"In *Hustle, Flow, or Let I* shame-free guide to rec own way. This book is tion, rediscover balanc celebrates your humani wellness grounded in the real world."

MW01200751

**Lara Love Hardin**, *New York Times* bestselling author of *The Many Lives of Mama Love*

"This book serves as a roadmap to a better life. Dr. Preston skillfully intertwines her personal journey with her professional experiences, meeting you where you are and gently guiding you toward a healthier, happier life. As a licensed clinical social worker who is also neurodivergent, I firmly believe that understanding how to make the world more ADHD/Autistic friendly is not only beneficial for neurodivergent individuals but for everyone, regardless of our life stage."

**Eric Tivers**, LCSW, ADHD-CCSP, founder of ADHD reWired

"This book is a lifeline for anyone juggling endless expectations. It's a powerful call to stop surviving for others and start thriving for yourself—authentically and without guilt. A must-read, it's not just a book but a movement toward healing, balance, and unapologetic joy that everyone should experience."

**Ana Maria Gaona**, former director of government relations and policy at the Department of Health Services in Los Angeles and founder and owner of Two Peacocks Travel

"In a world that has put hustle and urgency on a pedestal, this book offers a unique blueprint that will help you exit the rat race, embody grace, and find your true pace. If you've been longing to find what embodied wellness uniquely looks like for you, diving into the pages of this book is the adventure you've been awaiting."

**Xavier Dagba**, integrative life coach, shadow integration specialist, and author of *Scars of Gold* (forthcoming)

"Dr. Preston uses the totality of her professional expertise and alchemizes her own life experiences to offer this gift to the world. This book is a balm for navigating troubled times in the present and future, both individually and as a collective."

**Rahiel Tesfamariam**, author of *Imagine Freedom*

"*Hustle, Flow, or Let It Go?* is the perfect book for busy professionals who are tired of making promises to create more balance in their lives only to once again find themselves disappointed and disconnected from the flow they know they need and deserve. In Dr. Portia Preston's new work, she guides readers through the ways in which our to-do lists make us lose sight of who we are, reminding us of our purpose, yes, but more importantly, of the safe and quiet space within us all where we get to be our freest, messiest, most daring selves."

**Kristen McGuiness**, bestselling author of *51/50* and
*Live Through This* and publisher of Rise Books

"What a wise and unique approach to wellness! I devoured this book. Dr. Preston's kindness and personal experience shine through, wrapping her fresh and deeply useful ideas in a transmission of love. You will want to try her ideas and change what isn't working for you because you will feel so seen and cared for."

**Jennifer Louden**, author of *The Woman's Comfort Book*
and *Why Bother?*

"Finding your way to flow is not always intuitive or easy, and moreover, knowing when to 'let it go' can be as fun as pushing a boulder uphill with rocks in your shoe. This book offers a roadmap and credible tools to not only level the playing field but also help you get to that place where you are clear on the 'art of the possible.'"

**Awah Teh**, former chief data architect
of Verizon Media Group

"At sixty-seven years old, I thought I was already wise to the 'hustle' and had learned the lesson of 'go with the flow or let it go' by now. After reading this book, I realize these matters are quite complex. Dr. Preston writes in a conversational style as if she's your best friend, sharing her personal struggles while challenging you, through the exercises at the end of each chapter, toward self-examination. I wish this book had been available to me thirty years ago. It would have saved me much angst."

**Susan Hoffman**, former vice president of clinical services and
operations for Southeast Indiana Health Organization

# Hustle,
# Flow,
# or
# Let It Go?

# Hustle, Flow, or Let It Go?

### A Guide to Shame-Free Wellness That Honors Your Reality and Gives You Life

## PORTIA PRESTON, DrPH

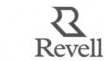

Revell

*a division of Baker Publishing Group*
Grand Rapids, Michigan

Published by Revell
a division of Baker Publishing Group
Grand Rapids, Michigan
RevellBooks.com

Printed in the United States of America

Library of Congress Cataloging-in-Publication Data
Names: Preston, Portia, author
Title: Hustle, flow, or let it go? : a guide to shame-free wellness that honors your reality and gives you life / Portia Preston, DrPH.
Description: Grand Rapids, Michigan : Revell, [2025] | Includes bibliographical references.
Identifiers: LCCN 2024054180 | ISBN 9780800772703 paperback | ISBN 9780800745974 casebound | ISBN 9781493445684 ebook
Subjects: LCSH: Stress management | Job stress | Mental health | Health | Well-being
Classification: LCC RA785 .P74 2025 | DDC 155.9/042—dc23/eng/20250404
LC record available at https://lccn.loc.gov/2024054180

This publication is intended to provide helpful and informative material on the sub-jects addressed. Readers should consult their personal health professionals before adopting any of the suggestions in this book or drawing inferences from it. The author and publisher expressly disclaim responsibility for any adverse effects arising from the use or application of the information contained in this book.

Cover design by Laura Powell

Baker Publishing Group publications use paper produced from sustainable forestry practices and postconsumer waste whenever possible.

25  26  27  28  29  30  31      7  6  5  4  3  2  1

For those who hustle
when there is no option to flow or let go.

You are worthy of rest.

May your wellness journey meet you where you are,
unravel your shame, and restore your connection
to everything you value—
most of all, yourself.

# Contents

# A Letter to the Reader

Our entry point to this journey is grace.

I glance at my desk, a graveyard of unmade decisions—some surrendered, others interrupted or never attempted at all.

It feels impossible to write amid the chaos of mail and scattered papers filled with abandoned writing ideas. Resisting the urge to sort everything, I decide to write from the edge of my couch instead.

*Didn't Maya Angelou write in a hotel room?* I do a quick online search to confirm.

I find an interview where she explained she didn't want any distractions: "I just want to *feel* and then when I start to work I'll remember."[1] I find comfort in knowing she, too, needed to escape her world to find the words.

*Surrender to ease.*

I repeat my personal mantra to myself, realizing that my body has confused this early morning dilemma for a life-and-death situation. We are okay.

The anxiety that made me feel as if I were attempting to jump out of my body subsides, my breathing slows down, and I feel seen as I read how Ms. Angelou describes her writing process:

> I try to pull the language in to such a sharpness that it jumps off the page. It must look easy, but it takes me forever to get it to

look so easy. Of course, there are those critics—New York critics as a rule—who say, Well, Maya Angelou has a new book out and of course it's good but then she's a natural writer. Those are the ones I want to grab by the throat and wrestle to the floor because it takes me forever to get it to sing. I *work* at the language.[2]

Ms. Angelou got it. It has taken years to allow what I have felt in my heart to find expression in words and make its way onto paper. Now, I have to embrace the imperfections in my own process. My brain struggles to find each word, concerned that anything short of perfection will not be enough. It says, "I can't do this. It's too hard."

Your brain may not work like mine. We are all on different journeys, but I'm willing to bet we each have our own stories of frustration and overwhelm. We recognize in each other shared experiences of pain. Here we can give each other grace to be honest about our struggles. We can help each other let go of what holds us back.

Sharing my story about my cluttered desk is an invitation into my journey. If I can embrace my own messy process, perhaps you too can experience the freedom of surrendering the mask of perfection.

I'm never going to have everything together. It isn't the point.

I'm great at a lot of things. But I still struggle—a lot. I bet you do too.

Sometimes, I feel stuck.

I have to be creative to navigate my roadblocks: a lack of motivation, decision paralysis, and the fear of failure. It's exhausting.

If I can lock into something I'm passionate about, I will give it my all as I forget my needs for movement, hydration, food, or rest. But if I'm not into it, I will do everything in my power to avoid it.

It took four decades for me to finally see my flaws not as failures but as a need for support. I could not understand the pain that lingered under the surface—a constant sense of overwhelm, intense internal pressure, rigidity, and the oscillation between an incomparable work ethic and avoidance of the simplest of tasks.

To the outside world, I was passionate, bold, courageous, accomplished. I seemed to mirror the "hustle" mentality so deeply prized by our society. For me, the hustle emerged through several points: the social and cultural narratives that compelled me to prize achievement above all else, the expectations of the academic and professional spaces I occupied, the need to survive in a world that lacks a safety net when you fall short, and my unique brain. It seeped into how I saw my worth and how I cared for myself.

> I have internalized the hustle as my method to success, so I feel safer embracing it than I do embracing rest.

But I'm getting ahead of myself. I'm eager to get into the rest of the book, where I'll tell you more—I promise. For now, I want you to know that you are not alone in your struggles. If I were to sum up my journey to this point in a few words, they would be these:

*I have internalized the hustle as my method to success, so I feel safer embracing it than I do embracing rest.*

If you can relate to this, I am writing this book for you.

Grace has shown me this is not the only way. It has revealed a different path, where I trade the hustle for a more sustainable approach.

As I write, I slowly explore the edges of my comfort zone, respecting the tenderness I feel. I start with small steps to make progress, adjusting until I eventually find a rhythm that works for me. I keep showing up, and one day I finish what I never believed I could accomplish. Then, someone turns around and says that I make it look so easy. And like Ms. Angelou, respectfully, I want to wrestle them to the floor.

The words I am crafting result from years of navigating the ups and downs of my personal and professional life. The lessons I have learned have taught me how to ride the waves while protecting what I value most. They have taught me to see myself as worthy, and to accept—not reject—my flaws and limitations.

*This* is how I summon the strength to boldly enter new experiences and spaces that terrify the part of me that wonders if I belong. *This* is how I forge community with others until I find the safety I need. And *this* is how I discern what comes next.

I want you to know that this is not where my journey began. We're going to explore the life I had before a series of health events changed it—where I embraced the hustle until I embodied it, and the pursuit of perfection seeped into every aspect of my life.

We will reflect on why I thought that was necessary for survival. And we will explore how I ended up here, embracing a messy desk as I write a book on wellness, hoping it will find itself in the hands of someone like me.

Someone who is curious about what is possible when we embrace our worth and lean into meeting ourselves where we are instead of where society thinks we should be. Someone who is determined to move forward with grace rather than shame.

Reader, you are worthy of releasing the hustle that has overtaken you and convinced you that you are supposed to be someone other than who you are at this point in your life.

You are worthy, period.

Join me at this shared table of humanity where you can explore what gives *you* life. You don't have to disguise, hide, or pre-clean your mess. As you read this book, remember you are worthy of setting the pace of your journey along with boundaries that protect you. Here is your permission slip to do what is best for you. If a topic or activity feels too challenging to explore, it is *always* okay to pause to reflect, sit with whatever resonates with you, and come back when you're ready. This experience is yours alone to create. I am here with you every step of the way, cheering you on.

Welcome to the adventure.

*Portia*

# Introduction

Shame-free wellness is for you if . . .

You were taught that loving yourself was vain and selfish.

You were taught to conform to others' expectations until you lost sight of yourself.

You were taught to express yourself in ways that were socially acceptable, rather than healthy.

You were taught to silence your intuition.

You were taught to chase external validation.

You were taught to value your body's appearance more than you were taught to meet its needs.

You were taught to pursue status-driven connections instead of genuine acceptance and love.

You were taught to abandon your soul's calling if it wasn't profitable.

You were taught to shrink yourself.

You were taught to avoid failure, even at the cost of your dreams.

You were taught to pursue perfection.
You were taught not to ask for help.

It is time to unlearn all of that. This journey is for you . . .

If you sense something deeper within.
If you're ready to take aligned, intentional action—without hesitation.
If you're prepared to push past doubt, naysayers, and overwhelm to live a fulfilling life.

This book is for people who have a love-hate relationship with self-help books. I am one of them.

I love the first few pages filled with promises, optimism, and hope. Yet, somewhere around one-quarter of the way into the book, I go from underlining phrases in the text to writing frustrated notes in the margins. As I become less convinced the author is human, I start to give up. Often, I don't even reach the end.

Instead of promises, let's start off with a confession: Early on, I thought this book would be titled *Less, You Can*—turns out I am the last person who should be writing a book on doing less.

The first part of my life ran on stress. In graduate school, I learned about how stress could negatively affect your health. I didn't believe it. I would soon learn firsthand how wrong I was.

A few years later, as I stood onstage at my doctoral hooding ceremony, embracing my mentor, Dr. Toni Yancey, no one could have guessed that beyond our visible commonalities—our race, gender, and careers in public health—existed a less visible similarity. We were both navigating complex health journeys. Dr. Yancey had recently been diagnosed with nonsmoker's lung cancer, and I had completed weeks of explorative tests and would soon be diagnosed with chronic kidney disease.*

*I will share more about Dr. Yancey's journey in chapter 2.

While my condition was not caused by stress, I was cautioned to avoid stressors that could worsen it.

This was probably not the ideal time to begin a career in management consulting. However, I had already accepted the offer, and my mind was made up. I ignored every warning sign my body gave that I needed to slow down. I pushed through increasing lethargy and leaned hard into proving I was worthy of this opportunity.

*Just. Keep. Swimming.*

It should not come as a surprise that my body was left with no choice but to take matters into its own hands. Within the first ninety days, I had a blood clot. I started to experience immense brain fog, and my pain and fatigue worsened. I ended up taking multiple periods of medical leave over the next two years. Every conversation I had with my team of specialists led to the same conclusion: The stress of my job was making things worse.

I reached out to a peer mentor I'd found through the National Kidney Foundation. I knew that she had a corporate background, so I hoped she could give advice on how I could push through without getting sick. Instead, she gave me the one answer I didn't want to hear:

"Slow down."

Did I want my identity, or did I want to live?

*Pause.*

I wasn't sure.

My goal wasn't to get well; it was to stay productive and thus worthy and relevant. My identity was rooted in my degrees, my job titles, and how others perceived me.

As a woman of color, this was a strategic move. There is a long history of discriminatory policies that have negatively impacted education and employment opportunities, wages, home ownership, neighborhood safety, and wealth of marginalized groups.[1] Even with an advanced degree, Black women earn less than White men with a bachelor's degree.[2]

Overwork was my tool of resistance. I wielded it to close the gap with each opportunity I was blessed to receive.

When we break through cycles that were meant to break us, we feel as if we are still on tenuous ground—never truly safe. With success, we enter increasingly exclusive spaces with their own hidden curricula and set of expectations. This keeps us always guessing and locks us into an endless cycle of proving our worth.

This invisible force drove my perfectionism and overwork.

I knew intuitively that the pressure I felt to present myself as capable and resilient had much to do with how the world treats Black women. Could I *really* admit that I needed to move at a slower pace? I was concerned with being seen as the four-letter word I worked so hard to avoid: L-A-Z-Y. The word I wanted to aim for was H-U-S-T-L-E. If keeping up a facade was the price of success, then I would perfect my mask: a smile that showed enthusiasm and comfort, a work ethic (cough: *hustle!*) that conveyed ease, and a strength that took breaks only behind the scenes.

For years, I alternated between sprints of pushing hard and bouts of debilitating fatigue. My body called out for a gentler path, but my mind was locked into the hustle. As a public health professional, I knew I was damaging my body by sacrificing it for my goals. Pushing through a grueling schedule to do it all and be there for everyone harmed me, but I couldn't see an acceptable alternative.

*If I do less, what will be left undone?*
*Will I be enough?*

## Success at Any Cost Is a Failure

Our society needs to have a deeper conversation around the factors that contribute to overwork.

Workaholism is an addiction to working that leads to adverse outcomes at the individual, interpersonal, or organizational level.[3] Researchers have found high rates of overwork among survivors of intimate partner violence[4] and childhood sexual abuse.[5] A study conducted among Norwegian workers found that workaholism was associated with attention-deficit/hyperactivity disorder (ADHD), obsessive compulsive disorder (OCD), anxiety, and depression.[6] Nearly one in three respondents who were classified as being addicted to work also met clinical criteria for ADHD, which can be worsened by trauma.

Our culture has shifted in ways that make overworking feel mandatory. For some people, there is an inner drive that compels them to work beyond their capacity. Work can provide a sense of identity, stability, and control.[7] For those who find refuge in their work, it may serve as a welcome distraction from chaos in other areas of their lives.

Among marginalized groups, the temptation to work beyond capacity can also be an effort to uplift oneself and one's community or to find stability and security. As one of few tenured Black female professors on my campus, my presence is evidence to many students of color that they can achieve the same, especially those who grew up in my home community of South Central Los Angeles. A student once told me, "Until I met you, I didn't know someone from South Central could do that."

While I am motivated by the thought that my presence can help students envision and fulfill their potential, I also recognize the pressure this puts on me. Many of our students are struggling to balance work, family, and school as they navigate difficult circumstances. They deserve our best. I have used this in the past as a justification to push beyond my limits to be present as a mentor and give my students the learning experience they deserve. However, not honoring my own capacity led to burnout.

By centering only *their* humanity and need for compassion, I neglected my own. In the end, this was a disservice to me and my students, who looked to me as a model for professionalism.

Success at any cost is a failure.

When I am overwhelmed, it becomes difficult to be patient and compassionate with myself and those I love. My rigid expectations go flying everywhere, and I "should" all over myself.

I know that I don't have to always say yes to every request or solve every problem. However, *knowledge is not behavior*, and the compulsion to push forward is indicative of a larger, more systemic issue.

## Behind the Mask

What hides behind the masks of the different titles we wear? What does our hustle conceal?

Are you the "strong" friend? The "tireless, confident" leader? The "one everyone can count on" to figure out a solution?

Perhaps you do everything you can to avoid letting others down—even when it means letting yourself down. Maybe you have tried stepping back, saying no, or delegating, but even if you succeed, something else comes along. Once again, you are stuck taking on more than you can handle.

As responsibilities build, tension mounts inside. You can't quite put your finger on it, but you know something isn't right. You're too distracted to pay much attention to the sensations in your body other than the dull aches and searing pain of working and worrying far more than you should.

Life is overwhelming, and there is no off-ramp for recovery. Anxious thoughts keep you up at night, or you wake up early with a racing mind. During the day, you struggle to stay focused. In your free time, you lack the energy to do things that you once enjoyed. The intentions you make to care for yourself shift to the lowest priority.

You go through the motions in your roles and deliver as expected. However, your confidence wanes as you wonder if others notice your mistakes and struggles with simple tasks. Do your loved ones notice when you are more short with them? How long can you go until you reach your breaking point?

You hope to find your way through this, but this time the path seems especially unclear, and your patience is wearing thin.

You want to return to normal—whatever that is. Where is the version of you who did it all? If you can't go back to that, you need to find a new way forward—and quick. You don't want to sacrifice everything you've worked so hard for.

This is deeply familiar to me. Because these are my struggles too.

My own wellness journey has been crafted out of a need to overcome workaholic tendencies and health setbacks. The intersection of my personal health challenges and my training as a public health professional allows me to use what I have learned to help others, even as I continue to evolve. Every day, I interact with people from every sector and walk of life whose dedication to their personal and professional roles threatens to come at the cost of their well-being.

In the classroom, I teach students who are often the first in their families to pursue a college degree. Many believe that perfection is the bar for success and question whether they have what it takes to succeed in the professional world.

As a speaker and coach, I help individuals to care for their well-being in the context of their reality, from high-demand careers to parenting and caregiving roles and the responsibilities of adulting. We discuss practices such as self-compassion to address harmful internal narratives that steep them in shame. We work together to restore their sense of worth and develop a wellness plan that is customized to address their identity, lived experiences, and unique needs.

We are all human and flawed, and the lessons we learn from our mistakes are critical for our development. I teach skills to help us all, including myself, navigate uncertainty, deal with challenges, and create more fulfilling lives.

It may seem contradictory for someone teaching sustainable wellness to confess they deal with constant overwhelm. Are experts even allowed to be human? Perhaps I should shed light only on the specific areas in which I do not struggle.

Spoiler alert! There aren't any.

My greatest wins come when I am willing to engage in the uncertainty of life and risk defeat. One step forward, two steps back. Progress is not a linear journey. It only appears to be because our society does a great job of stripping success from its context.

**My greatest wins come when I am willing to engage in the uncertainty of life and risk defeat.**

People see my accomplishments but not the circumstances I've had to navigate to achieve them. They catch the highlight reel but miss the private meltdowns. My calm and confident demeanor masks the pressure I feel inside. They can't see how often I am tempted to minimize my stressors, believing that privilege cancels out pain.

Although it seems there is an unspoken agreement in society to conceal our flaws, I can't afford to. I don't want to silence the pain because I know that when it is held in safe spaces and allowed to heal, it can be transformed into triumph. As I have shared my lived experiences with my audiences, clients, and students, the response has been overwhelming, leaving me with a sense that there is a hunger for greater transparency and reassurance that we are not alone in our struggles.

### Presence over Perfection

You are here because you are tired of responding to overwhelm by being hard on yourself and doubling down to meet expectations. You seek relief from this endless treadmill without compromising what is important to you.

Perfectionism tells us that our external conditions must be ideal in order to have internal peace. It leaves no room for uncertainty or flaws. It is both impossible and unsustainable.

The pursuit of perfection robs us of the ability to be present. Perhaps you can get away with neglecting your health and ignoring the quiet whisper of your intuition for a while, but both eventually have a way of catching up with you.

Protecting what you value most starts with honoring yourself.

Our wellness is at the core of all that we do, providing us with the energy and capacity to fulfill our needs and impact others. However, caring for ourselves can be a risky endeavor, as it is seen as contrary to social norms and the expectations others set for us. For example, my research on Black women indicates that the pressure to fulfill cultural and societal expectations of stoic strength and caring for everyone else hinders their ability to prioritize their own needs.[8]

The studies I have conducted on professionals in early childhood education and higher education showed that those who exhibited signs of the negative aspects of being a helper—such as burnout from the way their work was organized or traumatic responses to the experiences of those they served—reported poorer physical and mental health.[9]

Conversely, higher education professionals who reported experiencing more of the positive aspects of being a helper—such as finding meaning, purpose, and satisfaction in their work—were more likely to engage in self-care practices. These practices include mindful awareness, relaxation, self-compassion, finding purpose, and nurturing supportive relationships.[10] They were also more likely to report having supportive structures in their lives. This means that their environments—including the policies, institutions, resources, and people around them—were conducive to fulfilling their roles, managing workloads, and balancing internal and external demands.

When we have support and capacity to care for our needs, it is easier to be present, savor the good in life, and address what is under our control, even during times of struggle. When we are anchored in our values, we have more clarity about what to take on and prioritize. We advocate for our needs within our relationships, workplaces, and other settings. We construct boundaries to honor our capacity, understanding that our "no" is an intentional move to protect our "yes." These actions help to buffer the aspects of our roles that would otherwise deplete us.

When we honor ourselves, we practice compassion for all of who we are and what we have experienced—our strengths, our struggles, our flaws. We realize that our first responsibility is to respect and replenish our foundation. This has a ripple effect on everything we do: Caring deeply for ourselves influences our ability to positively impact others.

These are the principles I have used to develop wellness programs that have helped individuals shift from rejecting the idea of self-care to viewing it as fundamental to their well-being and satisfaction with their personal and professional lives. Through my talks with groups ranging from parents and caregivers to researchers and educators, I have assisted thousands of people in visualizing a personalized wellness practice. This practice is flexible enough to meet them in their current reality and equips them with tools to effectively cope with life's stressors.

Now I offer these benefits to you. By putting sincere effort into reflecting on your journey as you read this book, you can create a realistic plan to care for yourself amid challenges. You will develop the skills to address feelings of shame with compassion and construct healthy beliefs that affirm your innate worth. You will create an intentional and sustainable blueprint that honors *your* reality and is aligned with *your* needs and preferences.

This does not mean that life will be easier. I don't have the power to make such guarantees, and if I did, I would certainly start with my own life! This is about *detaching* from the expectation that conditions in our lives must be perfect or under our control. Instead, we adapt to reality by learning how to set our sails in the direction that the wind is blowing. The goal is not to be perfect, but agile.

This book is designed for you to go at your own pace. Some topics may be sensitive, and your emotional safety is a top priority. Since I personally struggle to focus when reading long passages, I have organized each chapter into smaller sections called mini-retreats. These mini-retreats delve into subtopics under each chapter's main theme and include reflection questions at the end.

I've also included more resources, including audio recordings and worksheets for the reflections mentioned throughout this book on my website (PortiaPreston.com) for you to refer to and use throughout your journey.

## Choose Your Adventure: Hustle, Flow, or Let It Go?

In our quest for success, we often lose sight of the need to care for ourselves. We believe that a time will come when everything is stable, and we can finally enjoy the fruits of our labor.

However, life offers no guarantees. Wellness requires ongoing attention and maintenance. This book provides a guide to three practices to maintain your wellness: navigating the hustle, finding the flow needed to thrive, and knowing when to let go.

### Hustle

Throughout this journey, we will expand our use of the term *hustle* beyond the scope of work. It will encompass any factor that hinders your wellness or makes it harder to care for yourself. This includes everything from difficult circumstances and unsustainable practices to a lack of resources such as social support. We will also consider harmful beliefs, expectations, and standards imposed on you by society, culture, and other sources.

### Flow

An alternative to the hustle is *flow*: the ongoing cultivation of your well-being and your connection to yourself, your loved ones, and the world around you. It involves adopting sustainable practices, creating healthy beliefs, setting realistic expectations, accessing support, and leveraging resources that help you care for yourself. The intention of flow is to enhance your ability to face challenges with resilience, build new skills, recharge your energy, engage in community, and live a fulfilling life.

### Let It Go

To shift from hustle to flow, it is often necessary to *let go*. Even when you recognize the need to change your approach or release something harmful, you might feel hesitant, stuck, or unprepared. Despite the warning signs, you may dig your heels in deeper because of the sunk cost—you've already invested too much.

This can take a dangerous toll.

If you hustle your way through forgiving, accepting, or healing, you will encounter even more resistance. So, we will focus first on what you are ready to shed, but we won't stop there. We will also highlight larger systemic factors that hinder wellness, such as insufficient resources and society's emphasis on productivity at the cost of your well-being.

## Our Roadmap

This book will guide you through navigating hustle, flow, and letting go in various areas of your life. In the first few chapters, we will focus on restoring connection to yourself, others, and the world around you—connections that may have been disrupted by the hustle.

We will reflect on your self-perception, your wins and struggles, and the thoughts and feelings that shape your behavior as you care for yourself, engage in relationships, and fulfill your personal and professional roles. This journey will equip you to create a personalized wellness blueprint tailored to what works for *you*—defined by *your* standards and values.

Every chapter in this book will guide you in identifying the source of the hustle in your life, finding the flow that suits you, and determining where to let go.

It is not realistic to abandon the narrative of living for others unless you have something accessible and practical to replace it with. To shed the shame that has cast its spell on you, you must cultivate a deep sense of love rooted in your worth.

## Creating a Foundation of Safety

As we embark on this journey of wellness, it is important to establish a stable foundation for your experience. Consider the following tips as you develop a safety plan tailored to your needs:

**Cultivate self-awareness:** Be present with your experiences, including bodily sensations and thoughts. Growth often requires stepping outside of your comfort zone. However, if you encounter significant discomfort, don't force yourself to push through. Acknowledge what you are feeling and assess your needs.

**Take action:** Identify activities that help you feel present or centered, such as taking a few deep breaths, stretching, journaling, meditating, or focusing on an object in the distance. If you feel overwhelmed while reading this book, allow yourself to pause, slow down, or skip content as needed. Consider taking breaks between sections to put the concepts into practice.

**Seek support:** Connect with trusted loved ones or professionals to discuss your thoughts and experiences. Reaching out for help is a strength and an essential part of your journey.

**Dig deeper:** Explore additional resources on concepts presented in this book that resonate with you and support your journey.

Revisit this section as needed to reinforce and adapt your approach as you progress on your journey.

This book aims to expand your sense of self by looking beyond the roles you play to see and care deeply for your own needs.

Throughout this journey, you will be prompted to reflect on your thoughts. Consider where you would like to capture your reflections, whether in a journal or using a notes or voice app on your phone.

Begin by setting your intention for reading this book. What do you hope to gain from this experience?

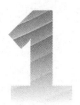

# Cultivating Self-Awareness

*A Bird's-Eye View of the Hustle in Your Life*

Perhaps, like me, you sometimes find yourself *unraveling*.

Drowning in an endless sequence of to-do lists. Grasping for hope while running on fumes. Struggling to care for yourself. We're accustomed to having a lot on our plates, but there comes a point where everything—work, relationships, current events— becomes too overwhelming.

We are all overdue for a retreat. The original definition of *retreat* is "to withdraw from." However, *retreat* is now also used to describe a grueling day of meetings interspersed with team-building activities. Instead of helping us to recover from life's pressures, we are encouraged to lean harder into the hustle, optimizing productivity while further exhausting ourselves.

For years, I struggled to justify taking the time for restorative retreats. I fantasized about where I could stay and what I would do, but never put my plans into action. It was only when I started to lose sight of myself in my busy life that I realized the truth: There would never be an ideal time.

The hustle will never slow down for me. It will never declare that I am worthy of rest. I have to declare it for myself.

Retreats are now a regular part of my wellness practice. They are vital to maintaining my sense of self. I have developed a few considerations to ensure they are aligned with my needs:

- I adapt my retreats to fit my circumstances. A retreat can be a luxury getaway that I've saved up for over several years, a weekend escape, a few hours in nature, or a DIY retreat in my home office or backyard that I can do anytime.
- I strive to be intentional about what I will do (and not do) during a retreat: rest to renew my energy, engage in my passions, embark on a new adventure, or reflect on my life and relationships.
- I consider how I can integrate the insights I gain from my retreats to better care for myself and positively impact others. For example, while I can't change everything about my circumstances, I consider internal changes I can make to prevent the burnout-crash cycle.

I believe that retreats should be accessible to everyone, even when resources are limited.

So, if you don't have a retreat practice in your life, why not start one now?

Refer to the sidebar titled "Creating Your At-Home Retreat" for a list of practices that have helped me design my own retreats. The best part is that you don't have to spend a lot of money or rearrange your schedule to make this retreat happen.

## RETREAT RESET

Don't you hate getting absorbed in a book only to be interrupted by life? I wish I could freeze your world long enough to give you the

## Creating Your At-Home Retreat

**Gather snacks and beverages:** Choose some of your favorite treats that are comforting and nourishing. My retreat menu often includes teas, sparkling water, fruit, vegetables with hummus, chocolate, and gummy bears.

**Find a comfortable space:** If possible, choose a quiet spot where you can reflect without interruption. If that doesn't exist, use headphones with a relaxing playlist to create a sound buffer. Bonus tip: If you really want to disconnect, disable your phone notifications. Grab pillows, blankets, or other items that support your relaxation.

**Set the mood:** Tune in to your senses. If you like scents, you might light a candle or use a diffuser with scented oils. I like to choose a music playlist that reflects my desired mood.

**Decide your focus:** The mini-retreats found throughout this book provide several topics for you to explore. Use a physical or digital journal or a voice app to capture your thoughts and reflections. Get ready to tune out the world, and tune in to yourself.

Modify these steps to suit your preferences. This retreat—this entire experience—is *yours* to create.

retreat you really deserve. While I'm working on that superpower, here's the next best thing: When you need to pause, use the retreat reset at the beginning of each chapter to ease back into your journey. You may use this section to recall what you have already done or reflect on your intentions as you move forward.

Now, take a few deep breaths to center yourself in this moment. What does overwhelm look like in your life? If you could find an effective way to cope with it, how would you feel? What do you currently struggle with that you could approach differently? Sit with any thoughts or feelings that arise before moving on to the next section.

MINI-RETREAT #1:

# TAKE BACK CONTROL FROM ENERGY VAMPIRES

## Retreat from Overwhelm, Uncertainty, and Other Life Challenges

Overwhelm and its life-draining companions are like vampires, depleting our energy as responsibilities multiply in our personal and professional lives. It can be difficult to cope.

Our self-expectations often mirror what we believe is the bare minimum: "I *should* be able to do this. I *should* know the answers." It is deeply frustrating when it feels like your strongest, best self is in the rearview mirror.

It's easy to think of others who may have it worse, but this does not invalidate our own struggles. These vampires don't discriminate—they feed upon us all.

Let's take a moment to tune in to our bodies with the following visualization. Imagine that your body is like a pressure cooker. As you take on roles and responsibilities, the pressure builds. Initially, the change is subtle, but over time it starts to take its toll. The pressure intensifies in your chest, signaling overload.

However, the release valve isn't functioning properly. Instead of a gradual release of pressure, it's either releasing it all at once or not at all. You experience this as overreacting to some situations while barely registering others, as if you were numb.

All your energy is diverted to managing this internal pressure. You start neglecting your personal needs and fall behind on tasks. The pressure continues to build until you start to lose control. You hold your breath, sensing that an explosion is inevitable.

Our bodies were not designed to function like pressure cookers. However, we are navigating a world that overwhelms us with stress.

It is *not* your fault. You are not lazy or unmotivated. If anything, the opposite is true—you poured energy into keeping things afloat until you eventually ran empty. Perhaps, like me, you have been here before.

Every solution you have tried to combat overwhelm began with the best of intentions to find balance by doing less. You may have experienced early successes in saying no, finding alternatives, and lightening your load, but life's pressures and distractions unraveled these efforts before they could become part of your foundation.

Even your best efforts encountered resistance. You found yourself reverting to a default state of overwhelm, with your pile of tasks seemingly stacked even higher than before.

It is understandable if you are hesitant to start again. Previous attempts may have fueled a negative internal dialogue about your capabilities or worth. To sustain change, the strategies you employ must meet you where you are, providing support to

- build a stable foundation that prioritizes your needs and values;
- address internal pressure to constantly do more;
- offer yourself compassion when you feel you deserve it the least;
- establish healthy boundaries that protect your connection to yourself and others; and
- let go of what is not in your best interest, even when it means disappointing others or embracing uncertainty.

The strategies we will explore will help you attune to your needs even as the world drowns them out, providing you with a stable foundation to navigate daily life with intention.

## REFLECTION

1. What practices help you tune in to your own needs?
2. Where are there energy leaks in your life (i.e., practices, circumstances, or relationships that drain you)? How does this compromise your well-being?

MINI-RETREAT #2:

# IT'S FEEDBACK, NOT FAILURE

### Honoring the Path That Led You Here

It is beneficial to reflect on past experiences with the understanding that they hold lessons that can help you move forward.

You had to go through everything you've experienced to get to where you are now.

Your past attempts to deal with the overwhelm in your life were not failures, they were *feedback*. They provide insight into what is not practical for your life based on the level of autonomy you have in your personal and professional roles, the resources you have at your disposal, your capacity to take action in the face of other obstacles, or the ability to say no or delegate.

These past experiences tell you what remains to be addressed. If a plan doesn't address your unique or less visible needs, how long will it last? For example, where is relief

- for those who are trying to survive,
- for those who are deeply flawed but appear to have it all together,
- for those who constantly seek control to ensure that they are safe,
- for those who don't have anything to fall back on,

- for those who struggle behind closed doors, and
- for those who wrestle with questions for which there are no easy answers?

Those of us who have hustled at the cost of our relationships, health, or peace of mind know that we can have it all, but we feel like we have lost touch with what matters most. We can simultaneously be on top of the world and feel empty and alone. We cannot achieve or earn our way out of the reality that life is not under our control.

Even if we "make it" on paper, our achievements don't tell all of who we *are*. The belief that life will be perfect once we have accomplished enough or fixed someone else's life will keep us from ever being free. There will always be something that falls short of our standards or expectations. This pursuit robs us of our energy and peace. We fail to see that even with every accolade stripped away, we are still enough.

On this journey, we will use self-awareness as a tool to bring into focus not just our past experiences but our current needs and patterns and the factors that influence our daily lives. This allows us to uncover a blueprint of what is feasible and sustainable in our individual lives. It positions us to explore options in the context of our reality without requiring perfection or control. Instead, we can harness our energy to make decisions that are aligned with our values. And that starts with honoring ourselves.

## Retracing the Footprints of the Hustle in Our Lives

For most of my life, I chased achievements and extended myself beyond my capacity to help others. I viewed my energy as an infinite resource that could be doled out in exchange for the validation I craved.

Over time, my email inboxes, text messages, and direct messages filled up with more requests than I could possibly fulfill. I

believed that my relationships were built on a reciprocal foundation of helping each other but never stopped to think about the
imbalance of only focusing on how I could give, not receive. I
hesitated to say no even when requests were not aligned with my
priorities because I believed it would damage
the relationship. I believed that people needed
me more than I needed myself.

**I believed that
people needed
me more than I
needed myself.**

When I did manage to say no or decrease my
responsibilities, it was often because I was at a
breaking point. I operated out of the narrative
that I should be able to handle more, rather than being anchored
in my reality. I only conceded to reaching my limit when my body
gave in to mounting exhaustion. In these moments, I felt stuck
and ashamed, as if it were a personal failure.

I was resistant to rest in all forms; I couldn't just sit still, take
a nap, or (gasp!) be alone. I was terrified of being left to my own
thoughts. I would fill in free time worrying about everyone
around me, obsessing about what others thought of me, or
wondering why I still wasn't happy. I had worked so hard that I
equated fulfillment with being busy or needed.

I felt safe in the narrative that the world I had constructed
depended on me, and without my constant vigilance, it would
come crashing down. However, seasons of depression began to
emerge. To the outside world, I didn't look depressed. I still went
to work, ran errands, and said yes to additional projects. But behind closed doors, I spent a lot of time alone in dark rooms crying,
wondering how someone who had achieved so much could still
feel like she wasn't enough.

These seasons taught me that this narrative was not sustainable for me. In the words of Jeff Foster,

> The word depressed can be spoken as "deep rest." We can view
> our depression not as sickness or personal failure but as a state
> of Deep Rest, a kind of sacred spiritual exhaustion that we enter

into when we are de-pressed, or pressed down, by the weight of the false self, the mask, the ego, the mind-made story of "me." Perhaps our depression is holy, and calls us to Presence, and contains the seeds of new life.[1]

Each time I experienced a season of depression, I wanted to return to this idealized version of myself who would magically find and sustain balance. No matter how many books I inhaled on slowing down or retreats I attended to learn practices of meditation and silence, nothing could prevent the eventual creep back into multitasking and the pressure I felt to do it all. This is where I would lose myself in yet another self-help book, only to emerge days or weeks later realizing that THE practice did not exist.

I told you I have a love-hate relationship with self-help books.

So, I set out on a path to redefine wellness in a way that worked for me. It couldn't require me to leave the hustle completely behind. I wanted neither to hustle until I dropped dead nor to embrace a soft, slow life in which I never experienced the thrill of a challenge. What I needed was the ability to act with intention as I dealt with the ups and downs of life.

I could move away from using the hustle to prove my worth, while still doing things I was passionate about—engaging in activities I enjoyed, connecting with others, and experiencing a deep sense of purpose. I could reflect on past experiences where I had allowed myself to operate beyond my capacity.

I sat with these patterns to understand how I could be more intentional with how I invested my energy. I embraced and integrated my experiences in a way that honored my needs. I found it empowering to realize that my own identity and experiences, from the culture in which I was raised to the values I lived by, were valuable guides in this process. I honored the wellness practices that were innate for me, realizing that dancing and singing helped me regulate my emotions. The "me" time I spent curling up with a good book was restorative.

I didn't have to shape-shift to embrace trendy wellness practices, but could adopt those that were helpful to my reality.

I came to trust that I was not defined by my hustle and that I was worthy of rest. My wellness practices became a foundation, anchoring me into safety.

What anchors you into safety?

Self-awareness practices help us tune in to and respond to our own needs, creating pathways to preserve our capacity and well-being.

## REFLECTION

1. Choose a past "failure" that you feel comfortable enough to reflect on. Looking at the situation now, what lessons might you carry forward?

2. Identify a practice that is not sustainable in your life. What needs should you consider when choosing practices in the future?

MINI-RETREAT #3:
# THE JOURNEY TOWARD SELF-AWARENESS

### The Road to Unveil Your Blueprint Begins Here

Imagine that you can take a bird's-eye view of your wellness journey to date. You've got a clear picture of where the hustle is showing up, where you are experiencing flow, and where you need to let go. You can also see how your unique experiences shape your journey. In this section, you will explore the role of wellness in your life and how it is influenced by aspects of your identity and lived experiences.

### Embracing Your Worth: The Foundation of Wellness

In our society, wellness is often presented as a means to an end, such as achieving an ideal body that will gain us visibility and acceptance. This ideal is typically defined by those in power. These unrealistic standards set us up to view our differences as flaws to be fixed. They become the conditions by which we reject aspects of ourselves and one another.

We are taught from an early age how to wield shame as a tool to keep our sense of worth at a distance, ensuring we base self-acceptance on our ability to conform to external expectations.

In the next few chapters, we will explore wellness practices that help us restore connection to ourselves, others, and the world around us. We will view each area of wellness through the lens of our inherent worth.

A strong sense of self-worth compels you to nourish yourself, advocate for your needs, and protect yourself from harm. It empowers you to care for others and engage with the world in a sustainable way. As we support each other in community, we affirm our collective worth.

My own self-worth provides me with a sense of safety to anchor myself to as I live out my values, embrace growth, and take risks. When I feel unworthy, I feel vulnerable, unsafe, and stuck.

Nothing makes me feel more unworthy than shame. I am not referring to the type of shame that has a healthy role—where our feelings in response to something we've done lead us to be accountable and take appropriate actions, such as asking for help or modifying our approach. This type of shame fosters humility—seeing ourselves in an accurate light.

Instead, I am speaking of unhealthy shame, the kind that attacks our sense of worth and hope. It's not triggered by something we've done; rather, it manifests as a persistent feeling of inadequacy, leaving us feeling perpetually unsafe, vigilant, and anxious.

It influences our behaviors and beliefs as a misguided means of self-protection—where the intention is to guard against failure, judgment from others, or harm by oppressive systems.

The belief that we are less than, too much, not smart, not attractive or successful enough, is not imposter syndrome—it is a defense mechanism to prevent the worst-case scenario. When entire communities have been harmed, it fosters a collective sense of anticipatory shame.

We think that if we do the right things, we can control our circumstances and remain safe, even though life is always unpredictable. Too often, we internalize the blame, and shame is the result.

Much of the hustle in my own life has been fueled by shame. It seemed like a reliable source of internal pressure to keep me on top of my game when motivation waned or fatigue set in. As long as it yielded results, it reinforced the hustle.

However, when this approach ultimately fell short, shame suggested a reliable place to cast the blame—myself. It taught me to protect myself from failure by taking fewer risks. It disrupted connection by making vulnerability feel unsafe. I believed others could not possibly relate or understand.

But I wasn't alone.

I blended in with everyone else who was nursing their own shame spirals, each of us alone.

This shame spiral is self-reinforcing by design. It is the result of a society that has wired us for shame by instilling us with the narrative that worth is derived from productivity, perfection, and status. This impacts not only how we see ourselves but how we show up in every area of our personal and professional lives. This spiral can only be unraveled by building a world that affirms our universal worth—one with systems to support, protect, and nurture us.*

---

*In chapter 8, we will discuss a strategy for how to address shame spirals as part of your blueprint for wellness.

We cannot do this without you, and we need you to be well.

So, this journey begins with securing your own foundation. Embrace this invitation to restoration as a process uniquely customized to fit your needs in this season of your life.

### Why Is Wellness Important to You?

Your wellness is your foundation for everything you do in life. During your journey, you will explore wellness in several contexts, including spiritual, mental, emotional, physical, social, your sense of self, and the roles or responsibilities you have in your family, workplace, or community.

You cannot sustain your effort to care for others or make a meaningful impact in this world if you neglect your own needs.

You might have relied on the hustle to make it to the top, but it was not designed to sustain you in the long term. When you focus on your wellness, you will become more agile and able to switch modes when needed. You will learn how to run your race at a sustainable pace, intentionally replenishing your energy and nurturing your mind, body, and spirit.

A fulfilling life can help you be resilient in the face of challenges. You will create the conditions to thrive—not just survive—when you are attentive to your needs beyond your roles—finding meaning and purpose in everyday life, maintaining healthy relationships, and engaging in activities that bring you joy.

Finally, your efforts to address one area of your wellness can have a positive effect on other areas. For example, focusing on your spiritual journey can help to strengthen your sense of worth, which in turn may motivate you to care for your body. Engaging in movement may positively boost your emotions, and a good talk with a friend may help you reframe your inner dialogue.

## REFLECTION

1. What does wellness mean in the context of your life?
2. How can wellness practices help you protect what you value most?

## An Inclusive Approach to Wellness

Our experience of stress is subjective—all the way from whether we perceive something as stressful to how a stressor impacts our bodies. Marginalized communities are subjected to greater levels of stress. Historical traumas such as slavery and genocide affect the health of subsequent generations. Discriminatory practices such as redlining in the US have prevented communities from building wealth, affecting neighborhood safety, job access, and the quality of food and education.

At midlife, Black women are estimated to have a biological age 7.5 years older than White women. This difference is attributed in part to how perceived stress, poor diet, and environmental toxins can alter gene expression and cause inflammation in the body, increasing risk of disease. This can have a generational impact: For example, the egg that eventually became you was in your mother's ovaries while she was in your grandmother's womb, exposing you to *her* environmental stressors.[2]

Inclusive wellness considers the intersections of our identities, acknowledging how multiple forms of oppression based on characteristics such as race and gender intersect to drive inequity.

Every aspect of wellness is influenced by our life experiences. Reflecting on my identity as a Black woman who is neurodivergent helps me understand my unique needs and identify sustainable approaches to address them.

The intersections of your identity and experiences can provide valuable insights into how you experience stress, allowing you to adapt your wellness practices beyond traditional mainstream approaches.

As you review the following prompts, consider what contributes to the hustle in your life, where you experience flow, and where you might need to let go.

### Personal Identity

List key aspects of your identity (e.g., race, ethnicity, age, sexual orientation, neurodevelopmental differences, and abilities/disabilities) that impact your unique wellness journey.

### Roles and Responsibilities

List your current roles (e.g., parent, caregiver, professional, student, volunteer, mentor) and responsibilities (e.g., household chores, managing finances, other aspects of adulting), placing an asterisk next to those that contribute to a sense of overwhelm.

### Lived Experiences

List significant experiences that have impacted your wellness journey. These might include major life events such as the birth of a child, the loss of a loved one, marriage, divorce, or changes in your health, employment, housing, or financial circumstances.

# Accepting Your Intrinsic Worth

*Restoring Spiritual Connection
and Protecting What You Value Most*

What determines your worth?

In a world that may not always value us, spirituality affirms our intrinsic worth. It encourages us to focus on what unites us— our spirit or life force. Spirituality transcends division, creating space to honor and celebrate differences while laying an equal foundation for all. Its essence lies in helping us see ourselves as part of a greater whole.

Your worth is not determined by your identity. Whether you wrestle with finding significance in your roles or experience neurodevelopmental differences, physical limitations, lack of social support, or financial challenges, none of these diminish your worth.

You deserve care, dignity, and respect.

Spirituality encourages us to live with intention and authenticity. The Golden Rule, a foundational principle across many faiths, instructs us to treat others as we want to be treated. This principle serves as a guide to building a more compassionate world for all of us, regardless of specific religious or spiritual affiliations.

As I share my own thoughts on spirituality, I acknowledge that my journey as a Christian may not resonate with everyone. My aim is to be inclusive and respectful, with the hope you will take what is meaningful for your own journey.

We are here to love and experience life, not merely to achieve, assimilate, and accumulate. We are *worthy* of a hope in life that doesn't constantly run on fumes. Spiritual practices like meditation, mindfulness, and gratitude help nurture joy, hope, belonging, and a deeper sense of connection with ourselves and others.

We were created for *community*. Spiritual practices encourage us to foster relationships, engage in service, and spend time in nature. They call us to share resources and engage in collective action to create a more equitable and inclusive society. When we appreciate our blessings and treat ourselves and each other with love and respect, we honor the life we have been given.

You are not alone.

And you are worthy.

## RETREAT RESET

Take a few breaths, inhaling through your nose and exhaling through your mouth.

As you begin to settle into your body, take a moment to reflect on the past day. Can you think of something that you are grateful for? Even a simple example can be profound, such as life itself, the kindness of a friend, or the beauty of a flower.

Next, think of one moment in the past several months that gave your life meaning or helped to shift your perspective. It could be a conversation with a friend or a challenge you overcame. Last, think about the past year. What is one thing you did to be of service to someone else? How does it feel to recall these moments?

# RECLAIM YOUR WORTH

## Recognizing Your Inherent Value

I once asked an audience to discuss how they perceived them-selves and how others perceived them. One woman shared that the world saw her through the lens of her gender and religion. When asked how she wanted to be seen, she simply responded, "Worthy." The room fell silent, an indicator that her sentiments resonated with us all.

Who doesn't want to be seen as worthy? Many of us carefully construct our lives around this pursuit, aiming to have an ap-pearance, personality, or lifestyle that is acceptable in the eyes of others. The problem with this is that the bar is always moving higher.

We don't start life this way. We don't question whether a new-born baby is worthy of care. What if worthiness was seen as a static and unshakable quality of our existence that did not wear off as we went through life? Imagine seeing everyone, regardless of their position in life, as having equal worth. How would that change how you see yourself?

## A New Perspective

Imagine your worth as the sun, a vibrant light that shines across the universe. Like the sun, your worth is undeniable. Picture the sky as your life. On a clear day, the sun shines bright, leav-ing warm golden hues on everything its rays touch. Your con-nection to your sense of worthiness is strong, making you feel secure.

On other days, there may be some scattered clouds in the sky—these are the opinions of others or life challenges that are bothersome but manageable. You may experience some doubts, but encouragement from those you love and trust helps to re-inforce your worth.

On stormy days, the sky is heavy and dark with clouds as rain pours down relentlessly, leading you to doubt whether the sun is still there. Your flaws are exposed as the struggles of life drown out your sense of worth. It is difficult to see in the moment that your flaws are just parts of your story—testaments to your endur-ance and windows for grace and growth.

When your sense of self-worth feels diminished, it is only an illusion. Your worth, like the sun, is radiant and whole. Even when the sky is full of clouds or the moon eclipses the sun, it still shines on the other side.

When life is at its most bleak and we feel empty, we must sum-mon whatever we have to shift our perspective. We must speak hope and healing into existence, reminding ourselves of how we have overcome. Affirming your worth when it feels it has been eclipsed by your struggles is an act of great faith.

## Creating a New Narrative

Our worthiness is not up for debate.

If we saw ourselves as truly worthy, how might we navigate differently in a world that is run on external validation? How might we care for ourselves and use boundaries to protect what we value most?

Boundaries are beautiful. They help you be proactive and in-tentional about protecting your capacity and what you value as you engage with others. They help you discern where to say no or let go.

I am a recent convert to the peace and protection that bound-aries can provide. Growing up, I only thought of boundaries as a set of rules I needed to follow to avoid danger. I believed that having strong personal boundaries would be interpreted as being selfish and would cut me off from others.

Over time, I came to realize that being overly accessible and accommodating compromised my well-being.

When *Set Boundaries, Find Peace* by therapist Nedra Glover Tawwab was first released, I excitedly purchased a copy. A few pages in, I was shocked to find out that healthy boundaries took work to enforce. They were not foolproof. People could ignore your requests and even get upset with you!

Boundaries seemed to be an invitation for conflict, which I had constructed my life to avoid at all costs. So, I put the book back on the shelf.

**Our worthiness is not up for debate.**

A few years later, I came to a devastating realization: Even if I gave everything I had, I did not have the power to fix others. I had anchored my sense of self in being a peacekeeper and a fixer, and as that identity began to unravel, so did my hope. I wondered if my achievements even mattered as I inched closer toward the prospect of self-sabotage. If doing everything I could didn't fix the problems I cared most about, what was the point of doing anything at all?

Without boundaries for protection, I lost perspective. I sank into a deep depression. I isolated from others, and my sense of self became distorted.

Thankfully, I managed to let those closest to me in and asked them for help. My desire to heal meant I would have to develop the will to take up space and honor my needs. With the support of loved ones and mental health professionals, I found a small flicker of desire to care for myself.

With time, I was finally ready to accept that boundaries were critical in my life and worth the ongoing work and commitment to uphold them.

However, I could not set boundaries with others until I established a few with myself. I had to come to terms with how I was treating myself, realizing this shaped how I allowed others to treat me. If I was worthy of my own respect, then I was worthy of respect from others as well.

I stopped expecting my boundaries to function as magic spells to make others meet my expectations. If my boundaries were not honored, I had to be willing to follow through with actions to protect myself.

While I will always have a caring heart toward others, it is never an excuse for me to accept harm or to neglect myself. When I am tempted to do this, I want to return to these words: I am enough.

Repeat after me: *I am enough.*

Take in the following statements slowly, noticing which resonate with you.

I am worthy of care.

I am worthy of love.

I am worthy of respect.

I am worthy of peace.

I am worthy of healing.

I am worthy of trust.

I am worthy of honor.

I am worthy of safety.

I am worthy of hope.

These affirmations become our reality when we decide that what happens to us does not define us. We are not immune to change—everything from our bodies and our personalities to our resources and relationships shift as we go through different stages of life. However, if our sense of worth is based on our existence, then we are all equally worthy. Always.

How we see and value ourselves determines how we care for ourselves, as well as our ability to show up for others and engage in the world in a sustainable manner.

## REFLECTION

1. When you look at yourself through a lens of worthiness, how does your story change? How do you see your flaws and struggles now?

2. What boundaries do you wish to create or enhance to protect yourself?

3. What words of kindness and affirmation can you offer to extend yourself grace? Take a few breaths and notice the feeling of your feet connecting to the ground as you come home to the truth of who you are.

MINI-RETREAT #2:

# REVIVE YOUR SPIRIT

## Embracing Practices That Allow You to Experience the Fullness of Life

A central theme of spirituality is *interconnectedness*—the idea that we are all part of a greater humanity and that we need each other. Our shared humanity encourages us to reach across the borders that divide us to share the richness of our cultures and celebrate all that unites us.

Spiritual practices help us understand who we are in relation to the world and inform the principles that guide our daily lives. Spiritual practices are organized into four areas:

1. Personal: what gives our lives meaning and purpose

2. Communal: how we express our virtues, beliefs, and culture in relationships with others

3. Environmental: our relationship with the world around us

4. Transcendent: beliefs and experiences that go beyond the material world[1]

In this section, we will explore several examples of spiritual practices.

### Meaning

Meaning allows us to find significance in our lives, from the seemingly mundane to the life-shifting. This can help us process difficult situations by focusing on lessons learned or broader outcomes.

Earlier, I mentioned my mentor from my doctoral studies, Dr. Toni Yancey, who had been diagnosed with nonsmoker's lung cancer. Up until that point, she had a vibrant life as a medical doctor, professor, poet, and model, just to name a few of her roles. As a founding board member of the Partnership for Healthier America, she helped to guide First Lady Michelle Obama's *Let's Move!* initiative.

Even after learning her cancer was terminal, she continued to embody intentional living. Almost immediately, she sprang into action to focus on what was under her control, making the most of the time she had left. She married her longtime partner. She continued her professional work for as long as possible, giving a TEDx talk just weeks after undergoing lung surgery.

In the final year of her life, she secured $20 million in funding to continue her legacy, the Instant Recess movement, which had captured the hearts of everyone from major corporations to professional sports teams, inspiring us all to keep moving ten minutes at a time.

Dr. Yancey stayed as active as possible, often taking walks around her neighborhood. I frequently joined her for these walks, and we talked about life and whatever was on our minds. We were simply present in the moment, savoring life. When long walks were no longer possible, we would watch basketball and chat.

What gave Dr. Yancey's life the most meaning was the relationships she treasured with loved ones, which included family (she set a personal goal of celebrating her granddaughter's seventh birthday), lifelong friends, and, fortunately for me, even her mentees. In the end, she taught us several important lessons: to lead with dignity, to never shy away from a challenge, and to face even the greatest of adversity with grace.

In her final days, she permitted camera crews from Showtime to film her story for their *Time of Death* series. It captured her courageous journey to live, even as she faced her own mortality.

To this day, I cherish my walks and talks with her more than anything she taught me in the classroom or any book, chapter, or article we collaborated on. I share her story to reinforce that no matter where we are on our journeys, each day has meaning.

### Perspective

Put simply, our perspective is the lens through which we view a situation. An expansive perspective may consider multiple views, while a narrow perspective might focus on a single, limited view.

Growing up, I had the perspective that I should see everything in a positive light. While this approach protected my sense of determination and safety in some ways, it also made it difficult for me to accept painful feelings. I'd simply stuff them down and hustle my way back to joy.

When I began experiencing significant setbacks, I no longer felt like myself. My identity was anchored in being happy, positive, and grateful. My close friends also struggled to see me any other way. They'd remind me of my strength and ability to bounce back, believing I could figure out anything. However, I knew the utility of my bright side approach had faded, and it was time to stop sugarcoating my pain.

I had to adopt a new perspective and accept that bad things happen in life and will continue to happen. This took time, but eventually I found balance in remembering that good things would happen too. This renewed point of view allowed me to look forward to an uncertain future and helped restore my sense of hope.

### Faith

Faith is a system or set of beliefs anchored in something greater than ourselves, which offers guidance for understanding life and how it should be lived. This may or may not involve religion. It provides rituals to help us navigate significant life events, such as birth, the transition to adulthood, marriage, and death.

Practices of faith include prayer, meditation, fasting, studying sacred texts, and engaging in praise and worship, whether individually or in community settings.

For me, my relationship with God is the bedrock of my spirituality. This connection is my refuge from the chaos of the world. Here, I pray for wisdom, healing, courage, bravery, endurance, peace, and hope.

When I don't have words, I simply sit in the presence of God and feel, surrendering the burdens I was not meant to carry—worries for myself, my loved ones, and the world.

I receive a love beyond logic, which allows me to let go of what is not in my control. To let all things be alchemized for good. Even the disappointments and losses that linger in my tender heart.

My faith has endured many trials and periods of questioning, which allowed my beliefs to evolve. This deeply personal journey informs my understanding of the world and my assignment in it: To love.

### Service

Service involves sharing our resources (time, money, energy, possessions, etc.) to help others. It reminds us that we all need each other. Practices can include everything from helping a friend to service opportunities in your community and impact on a global level.

When serving others, balance is key. We should avoid both extreme individualism—the belief that everyone should be able to provide for their own needs—and self-neglect that comes with trying to fulfill everyone's needs to our own detriment. It's important to set healthy boundaries that ensure our own needs are being met.

We can focus on the talents, skills, and other resources we are able to contribute to the collective while honoring our own capacity. Each of us has a role to play in advocating for and constructing stronger systems that provide comprehensive support and quality services.

### Gratitude

Gratitude acknowledges the impact that people and resources have on our daily lives, and plays a powerful role in shaping our mindset.

Gratitude helps us experience positive emotions by noticing the small things. Examples include saying grace before a meal, keeping a gratitude log, and taking the time and effort to appreciate and thank others for the roles they play in our lives.

Over the years, I have learned to acknowledge the reality of my challenges while remaining in a space of gratitude for my life and the glimpses of hope I experience on a daily basis. Reflecting on the distance between where my journey began and where I am now has taught me to savor the small things. This practice has sustained me through many difficult days.

### Awe

We experience awe when we encounter something so extraordinary or magnificent that we must expand our lens beyond our existing worldview to fully comprehend it. We don't have to travel far to experience awe. We can find it in a favorite movie in which the expression of love between characters highlights the best of humanity, bringing us to tears. We might also experience it in a dance performance, a work of art, or time-lapse videos showcasing the vast beauty of nature.

When I reflect on all that I have been through, I am overcome by emotion. I know that I stand on the shoulders of a vast sea of humanity, each of whom has played their role in supporting me. I am blown away by the immense and expansive love of God and how mercy has flooded my life. I have inexplicably navigated through all my trials to arrive in a place where I still find beauty in this world and possess a courageous, daring level of hope. The healing I have experienced in each valley has only prepared me for the next mountain. This fills me with a profound sense of awe.

Nature also evokes a sense of awe in me. I have witnessed the majestic northern lights in Alaska, the forceful flow of waterfalls in Iceland, and the beauty of the intricately rippled cliffs of the Nā Pali coast in Kaua'i, Hawai'i. These moments of awe in nature have helped shape my perspective on humanity. Each individual is a unique facet of a beautiful landscape, each with their own story, inherently worthy by design.

### Values

Values are our beliefs about what is important in life. If asked to name what we value, we might mention the people, things, and experiences that are dear to us. If asked what values we live by, we might say things like integrity or honesty.

Values help us find clarity about what we will prioritize amid a sea of options. They provide an anchor as we make decisions in our daily lives. When we live by our values, we are less vulnerable to the opinions of others. We know that our "no" is not rejection but an intentional move to protect what we have already said "yes" to.

## REFLECTION

1. Of the practices we discussed in this section, which feels the most relevant to your life in this moment?
2. How can this practice benefit you?

# UNLEASH YOUR AUTHENTIC SELF

## Uncovering the Impact of Hustle Culture on Spirituality

Our society's strong emphasis on individualism overshadows the importance of spiritual practices that foster genuine connection, such as gratitude, service, and living out shared values. We are conditioned to focus on what divides us, rather than what unites us.

When spirituality is exploited for power and profit, the result is harm to individuals and communities. Service is left to patch up the gaps of broken systems, abdicating the responsibility of society to meet the needs of the collective.

When faith is commercialized, values are reduced to lip service, and practices become transactional with the end goal of personal gain rather than fostering spiritual development.

In the end, when we are disconnected from relationship, from the restorative effects of nature, and from ourselves, we lose sight of what it is to be human.

We lose sight of our own worthiness.

The good news is, we can take steps to restore connection and our sense of worth. This journey begins by exploring where the hustle shows up in our experience of spirituality, what practices help us to find flow, and where we need to let go. Let's unpack this together.

## Identify the Hustle

When we live out our faith according to someone else's standards rather than what is authentic for us, we are prioritizing their acceptance over our truth. This can be difficult to navigate, especially if it is someone close to us. The hustle of chasing after their acceptance may seem like the better option, but over time we get further from ourselves and sense a gnawing in our soul to live out what we believe. This requires us to be not only introspective but brave.

## Know Where to Let Go

The expectations that others have of us, as well as those we hold based on a prior version of ourselves, can be difficult to release. It's important to be patient with ourselves as we evolve over the course of our lives. While some people may not understand our journey, if we look closely, we will find others who are on the same path. Embrace opportunities for growth and ask for help along the way. Personally, I have benefited immensely from resources such as therapy and social support on my own journey.

My community helped me grant myself permission to live authentically. They helped me realize that the purpose of my existence isn't solely achievement or pleasing others.

You belong to yourself, first and foremost.

In a pivotal scene from *Beloved* by Toni Morrison, Sethe, a former slave grieving the disappearance of her child Beloved, says, "She was my best thing." Her companion, Paul D, corrects her, saying, "You your best thing, Sethe. You are."[2]

We are our own best thing. And we must let go of any narrative that tells us otherwise.

While we often introduce ourselves to others through the context of our roles, this doesn't capture the essence of who we are. When we recognize and value our own worth, we become capable of engaging with others and contributing to the world in a more expansive and authentic way.

## Cultivate Flow

We can't just let go of shame. For too long, we have used it as motivation to keep hustling for the validation and acceptance of others. To experience flow, we must replace it with something stronger: a deep sense of love and acceptance that is rooted in our inherent worth and reflected in how we care for ourselves. This is a lifelong process; it doesn't happen overnight.

My own journey toward allowing love and acceptance to flow in my life began with finding tangible ways to *create space* for myself. I redefined love, realizing it was impossible to love others as myself if I did not first love myself. So, my self-love had to be the example and inspiration for how I loved others.

This was groundbreaking.

Suddenly, I *mattered*. My world opened up. I was no longer confined to only justifying caring for myself if it did not detract from my ability to serve others.

The same is true for you.

You *matter*.

## REFLECTION

Now, let's reflect on how you can do this in your own life: Identify the hustle, cultivate flow, and find where to let go. Remember to use your unique lens to answer these questions. That is, incorporate aspects of your identity, lived experiences, and other factors that you feel are significant in these parts of your journey. Also, consider relevant expectations, standards, or assumptions from society, culture, and other sources.

1. In what ways has the hustle—defined as unsustainable practices, inadequate resources or support, expectations or assumptions, or other barriers—negatively impacted your spiritual wellness?

2. What practices can help you to cultivate flow in your spirituality?

3. Where can you let go? Focus on factors that are under your control, and acknowledge those that must be addressed at the collective level.

## An Inclusive Approach to Wellness

Much of my spiritual journey has been nurtured through interactions with others. I have learned a great deal from those who share my faith through communal prayer, worship, and service. They have been a constant source of support, helping to strengthen my faith during challenging times.

I also have built strong relationships with people from diverse spiritual backgrounds. Our conversations about our journeys have helped to foster a deeper understanding of our personal beliefs as well as honor and respect for one another.

An ongoing part of my spiritual journey is cultivating my character strengths. I have found that in my work with professionals and students, character strengths are a tangible way for us to discuss living with intention.

We have the capacity to enrich each other's life journeys by leveraging our resources and strengths. Reflect for a moment on what you would consider to be your character strengths (see the sidebar titled "Identifying Character Strengths" for some examples). These are positive qualities of your personality that translate your values into action. Start by identifying a few traits that you believe you are currently strong in. Consider where they show up in your life. Next, identify a few you think would be helpful to develop as you continue with your journey.

I know it is hard for some of us to acknowledge our strengths. If you come from a culture or background that discourages you from bragging, or where putting the focus on yourself would make you a target, you may have learned it was safer not to stand out. You may have been taught that humility is not drawing attention to yourself. However, humility as a character strength encourages you to see yourself as you truly are, not as a diminished sense of yourself. So, you don't need to be so quick to lead with your weaknesses. Consider that you possess all of the character strengths in some amount, and we all have areas in which we can improve.

I consider some of my strengths to be love, curiosity, gratitude, honesty, love of learning, kindness, social intelligence, and spirituality. Each of these are expressed in different areas of my life. Love, kindness, and social intelligence show up in my relationships. I tap into curiosity and love of learning for the work that I do and to grow as an individual. Honesty, spirituality, and gratitude are vital for my personal journey.

## Identifying Character Strengths

The VIA Institute of Character identifies twenty-four character strengths organized into six different virtues: wisdom, courage, humanity, justice, temperance, and transcendence.[3] *Virtues* refer to aspects of our character that reflect a moral standard, prioritizing what benefits our collective humanity, not solely what is best for us as individuals. Within each virtue, *character strengths* represent positive qualities of our personality that inform how we think, believe, and act. Simply put, they are our values in action. Below is a list of each virtue and its corresponding character strengths.

- **Wisdom:** creativity, curiosity, judgment, love of learning, perspective
- **Courage:** bravery, perseverance, honesty, zest
- **Humanity:** love, kindness, social intelligence
- **Justice:** teamwork, fairness, leadership
- **Temperance:** forgiveness, humility, prudence, self-regulation
- **Transcendence:** appreciation of beauty and excellence, gratitude, hope, humor, spirituality

We all possess these strengths to some extent. We may be stronger in some areas than others, but the good news is that they can all be developed. I like to think of my character strengths as the catalyst to living with intention.

Areas I would like to continue to grow in include kindness (toward myself), honesty (communicating my needs), leadership (becoming better at delegating and standing in my expertise), and perseverance (not giving up on my dreams). At the same time, I affirm the work I have done to be more at ease as a leader, to persevere without resorting to internal pressure, and to be kind toward myself by slowing down and letting others know when I'm at capacity.

What areas would you define as strengths for you, and where do they show up?

What areas are you hoping to further develop, and how do you hope they will impact your life?

You can gain a broader perspective of your strengths by reaching out to people you know well. Share this list of strengths with someone whose opinion you respect and trust. Ask them to provide feedback on the strengths they recognize in you, along with examples.

If they are willing, invite them to complete the same exercise, and offer your feedback in return. Consider how you perceive each other's strengths. How are they similar or different? How do you each benefit from one another's strengths? This exercise illustrates the value of having a community where each person has unique strengths that contribute richly to the experiences of all.

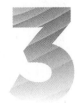

# Exploring Your Thoughts

*Your Inner World, Part 1*

Take a moment to imagine yourself in the following experience.

You stand at the entrance of a circular labyrinth whose path is hidden by thick bamboo and dense fog. Today the sun is not visible at all. However, just as our inherent worth remains intact, on the other side of the fog, the sun continues to shine.

You will enter the labyrinth at the outer edge and start to walk a path that spirals inward in smaller and smaller circles until you reach the center. As you walk the path, you will find that each of the mini-retreats in this chapter offers an opportunity to gain deeper insight into your inner world.

Along the way, you will learn tools to practice compassion for yourself and manage your thoughts and emotions. At times, you may encounter thoughts and feelings that are not easy to sit with. Remember, you are in control. Stay present as you work your way through the labyrinth, noticing how you feel. Consider your safety and comfort as you decide which topics you would like to explore at this time and which you may need more time and support to revisit.

There is no right or wrong way to do this. This labyrinth is designed for your unique experience.

The next two chapters contain a total of five mini-retreats that are designed to help you understand the relationship between your thoughts, emotions, and feelings, and how they influence your behavior. These chapters are presented together to acknowledge the overlap in these topics.

## A Few Definitions

Let's review a few common terms, just to ensure we have one central definition and understanding for each of them on this journey.

**Thinking:** The act of processing information or interpreting situations through the lens of your ideas, beliefs, and values. Elements of your brain and how it functions influence how you think, as do your past experiences and environment. Thus, the way you think is unique to you.

**Emotion:** A sensation in your body that is triggered by an internal or external experience, such as a memory, event, person, place, or object. You may feel increased activity in various body parts, such as your chest, head, or throat. You might experience a corresponding facial expression, such as a smile or laughter in the case of a positive emotion.

**Feeling:** The combination of emotion and the story created by your mind using your thoughts and past experiences to interpret the emotion, providing it with meaning. It is possible to experience a wide range of feelings in response to a specific emotion.

Our aim is to accept where we are without judgment—letting go of the habit of shaming ourselves for our flaws or for lacking sufficient willpower and motivation. Instead, we will explore strategies that will help us take a more compassionate approach, honoring and addressing our authentic needs as we move forward.

It is rare that we get an opportunity to reflect upon not just what we think, feel, and do, but *why*. As you navigate this material, it is possible that you might learn something about yourself that you want to explore further. While this journey will expose you to a wide range of tools and strategies, it is not meant to be comprehensive—these topics and our experiences with them are ever-evolving. I encourage you to take your time, as this information has the potential to impact how you approach caring for yourself and many other aspects of your life.

Near the end of chapter 4, you will identify what is contributing to your hustle, where you need to let go, and how you can cultivate flow for your inner world.

You are not alone on this journey. As a reminder that we all struggle with our thoughts and feelings, I'll be sharing some of my own experiences along the way. While we each travel different paths, our common goal is to identify our authentic needs and gain a stronger perspective on our life journeys.

## My Inner World

I wrote this book in a complex season of my life that shifted my perspective on each topic presented in this book. A work-life rhythm that had been invigorating became a hustle as I navigated new challenges. While I had occasional experiences of brain fog and fatigue dating back to my initial kidney disease diagnosis, concerning new patterns had emerged.

I was experiencing significant challenges with impulsivity and reactiveness, short-term memory, focus when reading and writing, and logical thinking. Tasks that were easily completed within hours or days just six months prior suddenly took much longer or were left unfinished.

This was a difficult time to be compassionate with myself, as these challenges coincided with increased professional responsibility and significant losses in my personal life.

The practices I had developed did not go far enough to meet the new shores to which my shame and self-loathing had expanded.

As the pressure I put on myself mounted, I was increasingly reluctant to carry out the simplest of tasks. I felt as if I was witnessing the erosion of my skills and, as a result, my confidence began to wane.

I initially was terrified by the thought of continuing to teach, speak, and coach in this capacity. Although each of these roles fed me greatly, I could not help but feel like a fraud in spaces where others appeared to have mastered all their struggles.

The only expertise I could offer was relentless curiosity and a promise that I would push through the new challenges that tested my entire body of work to date.

The best thing I could do for my existing students, clients, and audiences was allow them to see my determination, bravery, and courage in the face of uncertainty. I was discerning about which experiences I shared, careful to protect my own privacy and inner trust, and mindful of professional and ethical considerations.

To my surprise, the organizations I worked with during this time were grateful for my transparency and excited to have me share my story. My coaching clients found comfort in knowing that I was with them in the trenches, navigating my own struggles. My students felt that I was more relatable and that I respected the complexity of their lives outside of school.

And, reader, it is my hope that the vulnerability I've shown makes you feel seen and validated in your experiences as well.

This came on the heels of an adrenaline-rushed chapter of my life in which I earned tenure at my university and experienced sharp growth in my business. I had to slow down in order to preserve myself.

Whatever the prevailing wisdom was in achieving success and living your best life, I felt like I was doing the opposite. Deep inside, I knew the greatest gift I could give myself was the scaling down of my external commitments, allowing my needs to take center stage. I researched every angle to understand the rapid decline I was experiencing.

Finally, I found answers to many questions I had about myself, as the unique juxtaposition of my strengths and struggles culminated in a late diagnosis of ADHD and Autism. These two neuro-developmental differences coexist in my brain, complementing, obscuring, and challenging each other in unpredictable ways.

My seemingly extroverted, confident persona masked intense feelings of impostor syndrome and a deep need for solitude and introspection. My spontaneity and strong sense of adventure made it difficult to reconcile my struggles with switching contexts and going from one task to the next. I was a curious listener, yet I frequently interrupted others and missed social cues.

I was open-minded and accepting of others but rigid with myself. I followed rules but resisted and questioned those I did not understand or believed were unfair or unnecessary. I both needed structure and rebelled against it. To the outside eye, I was successful in achieving many challenging goals. However, behind the scenes, I put in enormous effort to overcome my own inertia. I was a speaker who loved to connect with and encourage others, but it took increasingly more energy to do so, and I required more space between engagements to prepare and recover.

I can only describe the months that followed as verklempt: full of every type of emotion as I tried to relearn myself. I feared that the legitimacy of my diagnosis would be questioned by many who'd known me for a lifetime by my masks. Learning new vocabulary—such as *executive dysfunction* and *meltdowns* and *shutdowns*—helped to erase some of my judgments, upgrading my perceived flaws and limitations to needs. Gradually, I was able to appreciate all I had done while unconscious of the heavy burden of the masks I had worn in personal and professional spaces.

In order to avoid burnout, I realized I would have to change how I approached all areas of my life. This involved redefining the boundaries of my relationships, roles, and commitments. I could no longer be the peacekeeper and problem solver, as these roles increasingly demanded self-sacrifice.

I am mindful of and deeply grateful for the support that allowed me to prioritize and address my needs during this time, from my loved ones and the health care benefits that provided access to medication and providers, to the autonomy and flexibility of my professional role. As I began to adjust to my reality, I recognized the opportunity to leverage my platforms to be an advocate for and to amplify the voices of others like me.

However, I first needed to do the inner work to address my own limiting beliefs. Only then could I fully accept that my gifts were not eclipsed by my challenges.

## Anchoring in Your Personal Journey

In the sections that follow, you are invited to reflect on patterns related to how you think, feel, and act. It's important to consider how they might be informed by any of the following factors:

- your social identity (race, ethnicity, gender identity, sexual orientation, culture, disabilities and abilities, beliefs, values, etc.)
- societal expectations or ideals
- your relationships with peers, family, and others (whether a source of support or stress)
- your responsibilities in your family, workplace, or community

- your access to resources and opportunities based on socioeconomic status, education, and so on
- your past experiences (major life events, traumatic experiences, etc.)
- Your mindset (the extent to which you believe you have control over the ability to improve your skills or make progress)

For example:

*Societal ideals*: I have internalized high expectations set by the educational settings and workplaces I have been a part of.

*The intersection of my race and gender*: A popular refrain in Black culture is that you must work twice as hard in order to be seen as half as good. I have internalized this deeply. It is harmful because there is no defined endpoint where one is guaranteed safety. It's designed to keep you on your toes. "Twice as hard" might as well be replaced with "infinitely harder."

At the same time, as a Black woman, I have been conditioned to mask my true emotions, modeling strength and grace under pressure. I am mindful of how easily anger and irritability can be weaponized against me. Thus, I may appear calm to others even when I am very upset. This is not only a strategy for success but sometimes a matter of survival.

*Disability*: My brain functions differently, which can make certain aspects of life more challenging. I grapple with internalized ableism, judging myself based on what I *should* be capable of rather than acknowledging my reality and embracing the support I need. This journey toward acceptance has a steep learning curve that requires time and patience.

Take a moment to identify a few personal characteristics that will be important to consider as you embark on this journey.

**RETREAT RESET** for Chapters 3 and 4

Take several breaths at a pace that is natural and comfortable for you. Pay attention to the rise and fall of your breath as you inhale and exhale.

Observe any thoughts that are present in your mind right now. You don't have to do anything with them; simply notice them. You might reflect on the nature of each thought—for example, an idea; a recent memory; an upcoming task; something you recently heard; or a familiar sound, sight, or scent.

Describe how you feel in this moment. Take a few more gentle breaths before moving forward.

MINI-RETREAT #1:
# DISCOVER THE POWER OF SELF-COMPASSION

### How to Move from Shame Toward Kindness

The concept of mindful self-compassion is rooted in principles that have guided humanity for thousands of years.* *Mindfulness* is the practice of being present in this moment, aware of your thoughts and feelings without subjecting them to judgment. The root of *compassion* is the ability to be present with others in their suffering.

*Self-compassion* is the practice of turning toward ourselves when we are facing difficulty, rather than abandoning ourselves or neglecting or suppressing our needs. Mindful self-compassion consists of three practices: *mindfulness, common humanity,* and *self-kindness.*[1]

---

*These concepts were first recorded in religious and philosophical texts in ancient India (Hinduism and Jainism) and early Buddhism, and are prominent themes in Judaism, Christianity, and Islam, among other religions.

This practice is helpful when we have a thought or feeling about a challenging experience and start to see it as definitive of who we are. For example, we might believe that we are unworthy of kindness or incapable of growth.

*Common humanity* refers to the realization that the pain we suffer in life is not unique to us but is shared with people all over the world. You are not the only person to make a mistake, experience a setback or rejection, or fall short of expectations. Without self-compassion, it is tempting to isolate or treat ourselves harshly.

By embracing the fact that we are not alone on the path of suffering, we can emerge from a downward spiral of beliefs. We might think instead, "I'm not the only person to make this mistake. I am human, and this is a part of my experience. I want to learn from this and grow as a result."

*Self-kindness* is the ability to treat yourself as you would someone you care deeply for. If someone you love made a mistake, how would you want them to feel? Would you want them to drown in shame until they had felt sufficient pain for you to forgive them? That is how we often treat ourselves. We judge ourselves, self-administering the amount of pain we believe is an appropriate punishment for what we have done.

When we are kind to ourselves, it doesn't mean that we are complacent. Self-kindness sends love into the source of our pain. This helps build a foundation for us to be accountable for our mistakes because we aren't compelled by shame to hide or make excuses. We can heal from the initial shock, take responsibility for our actions, and accept the consequences so that we can move forward.

## Practicing Mindful Self-Compassion

Here is an example of how I might use mindful self-compassion in my life.

1. Mindfulness: I feel overwhelmed with everything on my plate; I don't know where to begin.
2. Common humanity: A lot of people I interact with have expressed similar feelings. We are doing our best but feel as though we are barely keeping up.
3. Self-kindness: I'm proud of myself for doing what I can. I will try to focus on the next step and remember to take breaks to recover. Who can I ask for help?

Self-kindness can be difficult if your inner dialogue is honed to protect you from rejection or failure by setting perfection as the only acceptable standard. Sometimes when I make a mistake, it feels impossible to summon self-kindness. My knee-jerk response may be to speak negatively toward myself.

In a scenario like this, I'm my own demotivational coach. I will likely procrastinate or try to avoid the task altogether because I now feel bad about the task *and* myself.

In moments like this, it often helps to connect with someone with whom I have a foundation of deep trust and feel safe being vulnerable. I can call them when I am feeling my worst and know that they won't judge me.

They won't reassure me that I can figure it out on my own.

They will allow me to be human.

They will empathize with my pain.

They will remind me of my worth.

Slowly, my emotions will start to thaw. Gradually, I consider that their perspective may be more accurate than my own in the intensity of the moment. As suggested in the final exercise of chapter 2, our friends may be able to see our character strengths when we cannot.

The kindness of another person can help illuminate the path for me to shift toward self-kindness. I like to call this *community-activated compassion.*

Among my close friends, our shared history allows us to recognize the signs that someone may need support. We may not make a big deal about it, but we start to make a more concerted effort to reach out to that person. We will explore this and other forms of connection that can aid our wellness journey in chapter 6.

Self-compassion does more than benefit you as an individual—it creates a foundation for you to offer more compassion to others. Sometimes, we hold others to the standard we hold ourselves to. So, if we determine that we are worthy of being treated with kindness and give more grace to ourselves, over time, this may positively impact those with whom we interact.

Common humanity provides a platform not only for us to relate to our struggles but in all aspects of life. If we share in our pain, then we can also share in love and connection.

We can reinforce each other's worthiness and kindle each other's kindness and compassion.

If our differences can be used as a rationale for hatred, erecting barriers, withholding resources, and stoking division and violence, then our compassion and common humanity can be used to create bridges of understanding.

We do this for ourselves. We do this for each other.

## REFLECTION

Consider where you might currently incorporate mindfulness, common humanity, and self-kindness in your life.

1. Identify a challenging situation and note typical thoughts and feelings you experience. Keep in mind that these feelings are not facts, but rather the story you construct around your emotions.

2. Remind yourself that you are not alone in this experience or in these feelings. Think of someone you know or are familiar with who might have faced similar struggles.

3. Now, explore ways to offer kindness toward yourself. Imagine what you would say to someone you care for deeply if they were facing the same challenge. How does it feel to say those same words to yourself?

## HONOR YOUR UNIQUE BRAIN

### Breaking the Mold of Societal Expectations

Society has an ideal vision for how we should think, feel, and behave. We should be relentlessly positive, even in the face of defeat.

We should feel happy at all times.

We should never make mistakes.

This is not possible, as even those in the best of circumstances struggle—often with a different set of problems and behind closed doors.

A culture of toxic positivity requires us all to wear heavy masks.

The way our society functions, from our educational system to our workplaces, is based on a neurotypical standard. It is built on the assumption that we all think, learn, and engage in the same way.

**A culture of toxic positivity requires us all to wear heavy masks.**

When we think of people who have had major achievements, their success is a result of more than determination and willpower alone. We often cannot see the conditions that shaped their reality—from the opportunities available to them to their personality, support system, environment, resources, skills, and level of motivation. An inability to replicate success using the exact steps laid out in a book or course by someone else is often seen as a personal failure.

If only we had persisted.

If only we were stronger.

## Executive Functioning

Our brains are unique. Differences in how areas of our brains are connected are influenced by a range of genetic and environmental factors. These differences can impact our health as well as how we think, feel, and act. For example, *executive function* refers to a set of skills controlled by our brain that affect how we engage in and manage thoughts, emotions, and actions. These skills include things like planning, problem-solving, self-awareness, the ability to control impulses, and managing emotions.[2]

Executive function may be compromised in individuals with brain damage, degenerative brain diseases such as dementia, neurodevelopmental differences (e.g., Autism and ADHD), mental health issues (OCD, anxiety, depression, bipolar, schizophrenia), or substance use disorder.[3] It has also been associated with hormonal changes related to perimenopause[4] and menopause, maternal distress in the early stages of parenthood,[5] and PTSD.[6] It can even be affected by elevated stress and poor sleep cycles.[7]

According to ADHD expert Dr. Russell Barkley, when you experience executive dysfunction, it impairs your ability to determine

- what you will do;
- when you will do it and in what order;
- why you choose to do one activity among several options, based on your feelings and motivation; and
- your awareness of what you are doing, how you feel, and what is happening.

It makes meeting societal standards at any age a challenge, but especially the responsibilities of adulting!

I have spent years developing systems and strategies to help me navigate many of the challenges listed above. I think the hardest thing for people in my life to believe would be that I struggle to initiate or complete tasks. I've masked so well for most of my life that it seems like being driven is a core part of my personality.

The truth is, I do my best to lean into tasks that feel inherently rewarding. However, like many people with ADHD, I have more difficulty with things that don't provide immediate gratification. This means that my brain might find it more rewarding—and thus easier—to scroll on my phone than read a book.

I have learned so much about myself on this journey. For example, I must make tasks interesting and relevant, or else I will struggle with motivation. Understanding why I need to do something and having a sense of urgency helps me to persist through a task.

I also need to introduce novelty into my routines regularly to avoid them becoming stale and thus undesirable.

I now understand that when I am meaning to do something but find myself sitting and staring at the wall instead, I am struggling to switch between contexts. I need clear steps to transition between activities, and it can help to have something that feels engaging in the background, such as music, a video, or speaking with someone. I also benefit from reminders and check-ins to stay on track.

I have learned to recognize the signs that I am at capacity and take steps to scale back accordingly.

It might be hard to imagine that at times I struggle to pay attention, process information, or express myself clearly, given my roles as a professor and author. It takes a lot of effort and creativity (ask my editor!). I have benefited from writing coaches who helped bring clarity to my ideas. However, I still get swept up by perfectionism, relentlessly editing to the point where I must surrender what I have written. I trust it is enough to help someone, and perhaps its flaws help to convey my humanity.

I often lose focus and have to replay videos, reread a page, or hope I can fill in the blanks in a conversation or lecture where I have simply tuned out. While I have learned helpful techniques, they are not foolproof.

The greatest assets I have are also the hardest earned: patience and acceptance.

If I define myself by my mistakes, I quickly start to feel defeated, because I make a lot of them! I am writing this chapter with as much honesty as possible because I can only imagine how many people are holding their breath as they think, *I thought it was just me.*

It's not just you.

It is important to note that many of us struggle with executive dysfunction. If you can relate to anything I have discussed, I encourage you to focus on the symptoms that are relevant to *you*. Honor your needs and explore strategies or resources that might help you.

## Cognitive Distortions

Another challenge related to how we think is *cognitive distortion*. This refers to patterns of thinking, such as limiting beliefs, that are irrational or untrue. Distorted thinking can be hard to detect because it *seems* realistic to us. However, it can lead us to think negatively about ourselves or situations we're in.

Examples of cognitive distortions include

- binary thinking (seeing things as black and white with no room for nuance)
- focusing on the negatives while disregarding the positives (only seeing the bad in a situation)
- personalizing problems (thinking everything is your fault)
- solely blaming others without taking any responsibility (thinking everything is someone else's problem)
- diminishing your strengths or achievements (thinking nothing you do is good enough)

- believing others do not like you without any proof (believing everyone is against you)
- insisting things must or should go a certain way (not accepting reality)
- catastrophizing situations (assuming things will turn out poorly)[8]

I frequently experience cognitive distortions, despite having taught my students how to navigate them for years! Some of my struggles include binary thinking, worrying others have a negative perception of me, and envisioning the worst-case scenario.

Cognitive distortions are like fun-house mirrors, preventing us from seeing situations accurately. Here are a few strategies that can help you identify and address them when they pop up:

1. Listen to your inner dialogue. This will help you better detect some of your common thought patterns over time.
2. Reflect on your past experiences with cognitive distortions. Do you notice any triggers? What helps you work through them? For example, I tend to focus on the worst-case scenario if I am feeling a great deal of pressure. So, I try to challenge myself to think of other options for how the situation might turn out. If you're certain you will fail in a situation, you might ask yourself, "And what if I succeed?"
3. Explore your limiting beliefs. These are important to address because they can stand in the way of what you want most. What is at the root of your belief? Is it true? How might you address or overcome it? Sometimes, I convince myself that I can't do something because I don't want to face difficulty, criticism, or rejection. I try to consider if it is something I truly want and whether it is deeply aligned with my values. If it is, then it is worth the effort to do

my best. I would rather be denied after having given it
my all than reject myself outright.

A recurring cognitive distortion in my own life that appears in
everything from my professional career to my personal relationships is the belief that things should be easy and go the way that
I expect. However, I know that I cannot escape difficulty in life.

Sometimes, if I am feeling overwhelmed, especially when dealing with a long-term project, I decrease the pressure by allowing
myself to quit for the moment in my head. This is different from
taking a break, because it means I completely step out of having a specific role or responsibility. This brings me some relief
because it gives me a sense of agency. I came up with this during
my doctoral studies. When I hit my limit, I would take a day or
two to watch reality TV or visit the beach. This act of freedom
often let me cool off a bit from whatever was bothering me at
school. Now, we would probably call this taking a mental health
day. At the time, it gave me the distance I needed to come back
and approach things from a different perspective.

## REFLECTION

1. What have you noticed is unique about the way you
   think or process information?
2. What are some of your common thought patterns?
3. What, if any, cognitive distortions do you experience?
   How might you utilize the strategies in this section to
   help you address them?

## An Inclusive Approach to Wellness

Mental health issues affect one in five people in the United States
(23.1 percent).[9] They are more prevalent among women compared to men and people under the age of twenty-five compared

to older age groups. Of those who have a mental health issue, only half are receiving treatment.

It is estimated that globally 15–20 percent of people are neurodivergent.[10] Considering the unique ways in which our brains function and the mental health challenges many of us face, places such as schools, workplaces, and other settings play a vital role in addressing our needs and allowing us to participate in society in a meaningful way.

Strategies developed by the Centers for Disease Control and Prevention to promote mental health and well-being among students include instruction on topics such as mental health issues, mindfulness, acceptance, and coping; fostering socioemotional learning; strengthening connections between students, their families, and school staff; and addressing staff well-being.[11] The University of San Diego School for Leadership and Education Sciences suggests that schools can better support the needs of neurodivergent students by creating an environment that is psychologically safe, using additional learning formats beyond a standard lecture—such as hands-on activities—to teach students, celebrating a student's strengths, engaging parents to help determine how to best address a child's needs, and providing a consistent routine in the classroom.[12]

In workplaces, strategies to support neurodivergent employees include creating a supportive culture free from bullying and discrimination, addressing biases in hiring, providing support for sensory needs (e.g., lighting, headphones), adjusting social expectations so that individuals are not pressured to socially mask, and offering remote or hybrid work options and flexible scheduling so that individuals can work when they are most productive.[13] We will discuss workplace strategies to address mental health in chapter 7.

When adequate support is not provided, it can severely impact one's well-being. For example, many Autistics struggle to participate in the workforce, which greatly impacts their quality of life and ability to fulfill basic needs.

Many people have referred to Autistics and other under-resourced populations as canaries in the coal mine of society. Miners often took canaries with them into coal mines because of these birds' sensitivity to hazardous conditions, including the presence of deadly carbon monoxide. If the bird collapsed or showed signs of distress, it served as an early warning signal to the miners of imminent danger, cautioning them to exit the mine. Similarly, vulnerable populations are the first to be impacted by systemic failures. Being responsive to their needs helps to build a stronger, healthier society. However, problems that are not addressed become bigger, ultimately affecting us all.

We are strongest when we are united in our humanity, seeing ourselves in each other and accepting that our fates are interwoven. By working together, we can serve as effective allies for each other and proactively address critical needs in our society. This cycle of giving and receiving establishes a flow that deepens our human bond.

# Managing Your Emotions

*Your Inner World, Part 2*

Your focus returns to the labyrinth as you hear the gentle crunch of pebbles beneath your feet. You walk along a bamboo-lined path at a slow, intentional pace, savoring each step as you unlock more of yourself. The rhythm of your steps is the only sound you hear, and it has a calming effect on your spirit.

Finally, you reach the center of the labyrinth, where a Zen garden awaits, its gravel raked meticulously into rows.

As you follow the circular path along the garden's perimeter, you encounter stones representing seven universal emotions: anger, contempt, disgust, enjoyment, fear, sadness, and surprise.[1] These emotions arise in response to experiences and stimuli deemed important by our bodies. They may manifest as facial expressions, physical sensations such as a tightness in our chest, or behaviors such as laughing or crying.

Each stone marks a station for reflection. There is also a feelings wheel to help you describe your experience of emotions with greater specificity.[2] You recall that feelings are created when we interpret our emotions through thoughts or past experiences. For instance, the emotion of surprise may be processed as a feeling of awe, astonishment, disillusionment, dismay, or shock.

At the end of the path, there is a board inviting you to share what experiences trigger specific emotions and how you recognize them. You are asked to place a pin next to the feelings that are resonant for you. There are comments left by previous visitors discussing their experiences of various feelings and how they cope with them.

They explained how positive feelings, like peace, power, and joy, are associated with relationships, hobbies, achievements, and quiet moments of reflection. You get the sense that these feelings fuel their sense of self-worth and make their lives meaningful.

However, the other visitors left far more pins for negative feelings such as sad, mad, and scared. Here, people described experiences of uncertainty, conflict, grief, disappointment, loss, and failure. You think about the stark contrast between the two types of experiences, and how rarely such honest conversations occur in daily life. You take a moment to reflect on how you feel and add your thoughts to each board.

In this chapter, we will explore the emotions and feelings we experience, and how we are conditioned to express them (or not). We will discuss tools to help us honor and find healthy expression for a wide range of emotions.

Because when we habitually stuff down how we feel, it doesn't go away.

Our bodies hold these stories, packing them in tightly with tension, and they leap out in our interactions when we least expect it.

We have to find a better way.

## We Are Not Fine

Consider one of the most common ways we greet one another: "How are you doing?"

It's hard to tell if the other person is being sincere or just polite. So we typically respond with options that quickly end the exchange: "Good," "Great," "Fantastic," or "Fine."

However, the 2022 Stress in America survey reveals that most of us are not fine.[3] Three out of four respondents indicated that stress regularly impacts their lives negatively.

Imagine responding truthfully in a conversation with one of the following statements:

- **I'm overwhelmed.** One in three people reported they felt overwhelmed by stress on most days (34 percent).
- **I don't feel well.** Three in four people reported stress-related health effects in the past month, including headaches (38 percent), fatigue (35 percent), and feelings of anxiety (34 percent) or depression (33 percent).
- **I'm struggling to care for myself.** One in three people reported that stress affected mental health (36 percent), eating habits (33 percent), physical health (32 percent), and motivation for hobbies (30 percent).
- **I'm worried about everything.** Nearly a third of respondents reported constant worry (30 percent).
- **I don't know.** One in five people reported that stress impacts memory (21 percent), concentration (20 percent), and decision-making (17 percent).

If you were to use these responses with a family member, friend, or colleague, who would express genuine concern? Who would say, "You'll figure it out, you always do!" or "You'll be fine!"? Or worse, would they criticize you for opening up? How would that make you feel? I hear these all the time. And while they are meant to be reassuring, they only make me feel worse.

Stress profoundly affects our personal and professional lives. According to the survey, a quarter of adults feel so stressed most days that it impairs their ability to function (27 percent). More than one in three feel unable to take any action when stressed (37 percent). Recall what we just discussed in the last chapter about executive dysfunction. On days when you feel overwhelmed by even the thought of starting your first task, remember this:

You are not lazy. You are using all your energy to survive.

We are not all "fine."

The only way to dispel this narrative is through connection. Consider the words of Dr. Margaret McFarland, a developmental psychologist and a major influence behind the televised children's series *Mister Rogers' Neighborhood*: "Anything human is mentionable, and anything mentionable is manageable."[4]

So how do we move forward in community with one another in a way that honors all our experiences?

How do we acknowledge and manage our emotions in a way that frees us from shame and our own expectations?

## RETREAT RESET

*Welcome back. Your retreat reset for this chapter can be found on page 70.*

## MINI-RETREAT #1:
## FEEL IN ORDER TO HEAL

### Honoring Both Positive and Negative Emotions

Dismissive reactions to a person sharing their honest feelings reveal a deeper truth about our society: We struggle to honor and accept the full range of human emotions.

We are conditioned to believe we should be happy all the time. If we aren't, something is wrong with us. And there is usually a solution that can be sold to us in the form of possessions, money, or social approval.

We receive messages as early as childhood about which emotions are safe to express. In many communities, this imprinting varies across gender lines—girls may be socialized to show only pleasant emotions, and young boys may be taught to show no emotion at all. But negative emotions can provide important insights, such as when we need time and support to heal, when our boundaries are being crossed, or when there is harm that needs to be addressed or repaired to avoid irreparable damage. Suppressing emotions can lead to coping in a way that harms ourselves and others.

Today's society has few guardrails in place to protect our emotional well-being. We are increasingly exposed to media that can manipulate our attention by provoking fear without providing tools to help us process information, put it into context, and encourage civil interactions.

We lack guidance on how to effectively cope with disappointment, pain, and rejection. In our productivity-driven culture, emotions such as grief and persistent emotional states such as mood disorders are treated as inconveniences to the bottom line. Often, a failure to consistently deliver results is seen as a failure of the individual, rather than a failure of the culture itself. We learn to hide our personal suffering and compartmentalize, but how can this be sustainable? At a certain point, the cost is connection to ourselves and others.

Too often, those who have experienced trauma are met with blame rather than support. We fail to address the trauma at the source—which is often directly or indirectly the result of societal inequities. Trauma can have long-term effects, altering how we think, feel, and act.

It was only in recent years that I was able to understand my own traumatic responses to life experiences. With the support of therapists who used talk-based and somatic (body-based) practices, I learned tools to help me feel safe processing my emotions and experiences.

We cannot control our circumstances in a way that eliminates disappointment or uncertainty. We need community and ongoing support to navigate life's challenges, not just encouragement to put them behind us.

No one deserves hardship. Our tragedies are not fodder for purpose or inspiration.

While the insights you gain as a result of your challenges can foster growth and resilience, this does not justify what happened. Instead, they reflect your courage to face reality and integrate painful experiences. They are a part of your story, but they do not define you. Your ability to find meaning invokes light into the deepest of despairs.

**Daring to speak life into yourself and renew your hope is the catalyst that moves you forward, creating meaning in the wake of all you have survived.**

Daring to speak life into yourself and renew your hope is the catalyst that moves you forward, creating meaning in the wake of all you have survived.

Emotions serve as a compass, helping us understand and honor our needs. Positive emotions such as joy and peace help us identify the interactions and experiences that make our lives fulfilling. At the same time, emotions perceived as negative, such as sadness or frustration, help us identify where we are struggling and what we need to accept, change, or let go of in our lives. Other emotions, like surprise, might be considered positive, negative, or neutral depending on the context. Mixed emotions may arise when something reminds us of a loved one who has passed, evoking both joy and heartache.

And *all* of these emotions are valid.

It isn't always easy to be present with our emotions as we experience them. It can feel overwhelming when emotions trigger our body's stress response. However, we can learn techniques that help us move through the stress cycle and activate our relaxation response.

It's important to find healthy ways to cultivate positive emotions and navigate, rather than suppress, those we find more challenging. Developing these skills as an ongoing practice can help to ensure we are able to access and implement them in times of stress. As we develop agility, we can experience a broader spectrum of emotions, using their insights as a guide to help us move forward.

Observing how you feel when you experience an emotion can help you better understand your own patterns. A study conducted in Finland, Sweden, and Taiwan found similarities among participants across cultures when they were asked how their bodies respond to emotions.[5] For example, happiness sparked activity throughout the body, while depression led to inactivity. Fear, shame, and envy were associated with more activity in the chest.

I find it easier to detect positive emotions, such as joy, than difficult ones. This may be due in part to alexithymia, a trait associated with Autism that indicates difficulty identifying and understanding emotions. Sometimes I need to reflect on my interactions with others to realize I am upset, or realize that feelings of tension in my shoulders, neck, and back are cues that I may feel distressed.

When I am feeling upset, I might want to respond in a way that is not helpful. When possible, I try to honor my emotions by allowing myself to fully express what I'm feeling. If that is not possible, I might reflect on my own or with someone I trust to identify options for how I can respond. While it takes time to process my emotions, it ultimately helps me move forward.

I am often saddened by the state of the world. The news focuses on what is going wrong in our world, as that attracts more consistent viewership. I have learned to be discerning about where and when I access information, noting my emotions before and after. At times, I've had to distance myself for my own protection. I want to be informed, but not at the cost of my well-being.

It is important to remember that as you learn to honor your authentic emotions, not everyone will understand or be able to honor your experiences.

This does not make them any less valid.

You are not responsible for convincing others—this is about living in integrity with yourself.

## REFLECTION

Think back to the stations in the labyrinth that explored emotions and corresponding feelings. It may be helpful for you to refer to the feelings wheel for this reflection.[6]

1. **Identify positive emotions:** What positive emotions (e.g., calm, confidence, joy) do you often feel, and in what situations do they arise? How can you encourage more of these feelings in your life?
2. **Explore negative emotions:** What negative emotions (e.g., anger, sadness) do you frequently experience, and in what contexts? How might you better manage these feelings?

MINI-RETREAT #2:
# FLEX YOUR EMOTIONAL INTELLIGENCE

## How Emotions Influence Your Life

Some of us feel confident in our ability to manage our emotions, while others seem to be managed by them. While there are likely many explanations, one factor that makes a critical difference is emotional intelligence.

This powerful set of skills enables us to recognize and understand both our own emotions and those of others. It empowers us to make decisions and take actions that help us effectively navigate relationships, manage finances, care for ourselves, lead, inspire others, and live fulfilling lives. Finally, emotional intelligence helps us contribute positively to our communities.

Our relationships suffer when we fail to manage our emotions or understand and respond in an appropriate manner to someone else's. When we are overcome with stress, we may find ourselves lashing out at those we love the most, only to regret it afterward. Additionally, leaders with great expertise or skill are often hindered by an inability to relate to or positively motivate and influence their employees and those they serve.

Another factor that significantly impacts our ability to manage our well-being is our finances, as this influences the extent to which we can care for our needs and those of our loved ones. In a 2024 survey of a sample of American adults, nearly half reported that worries about money had a negative impact on their mental health.[7]

## Understanding Emotional Intelligence

Let's explore emotional intelligence using the Emotional Quotient Inventory (EQ-i 2.0).[8] This framework encompasses five key areas: self-perception, self-expression, interpersonal skills, decision-making, and stress management. I'll share examples from my personal journey to illustrate how each component contributes to personal growth and well-being.

### Self-Perception

Self-perception includes self-regard, self-actualization, and emotional self-awareness.

For me, developing a healthy sense of self-regard involves maintaining steady confidence and respect for myself, even when I make mistakes. My identity isn't defined solely by my strengths or weaknesses.

I once viewed self-actualization as a peak to be reached and maintained through hard work. However, I learned it's about intentionally pursuing meaningful growth and development as part of a fulfilling life. Despite our best efforts, all life journeys have ups and downs.

Of these skills, emotional self-awareness was the hardest for me to embrace. When I am triggered by a situation, it can provoke intense emotion that sends me spiraling. I feel reactionary and lose control of my emotions. It took years to learn how to respond in these situations.

I now identify my emotions and try to understand their roots, considering how they affect me and those around me. This awareness helps me recognize my typical stress response patterns:

In **fight mode**, I become defensive, and my perspective is narrow.

In **flight mode**, I avoid the stressor at all costs.

In **freeze mode**, I'm unable to do or process anything.

In **fawn mode**, I overlook my own needs to please others.

Embracing my emotions took bravery. I used to escape or suppress them because I was convinced that they would overtake me. However, I have now developed the ability to feel so that I can heal.

My emotions offer important clues to addressing my needs so I can move forward. Feelings of tenderness or tension help me know when to pause, set a boundary, or take a stand. Taking time to reflect on how I feel can help me process my emotions, building trust with my body that I will take the appropriate action to care for its needs.

### Self-Expression

Self-expression includes emotional expression, assertiveness, and independence.

I experience emotions intensely, so my reactions to feeling un-heard, misunderstood, or disrespected can sometimes seem over the top. When possible, I slow down and use tools for healthy emotional expression, considering the best words, tone, and cues to effectively convey my feelings. I wish I'd had these tools in my twenties—they would have made communication in relation-ships much easier!

When having important conversations, in-person interac-tions include nuance through verbal and nonverbal cues that text and email lack. A smile or raised voice offers insight into what the other person feels and what the most appropriate re-sponse would be.

I have noticed that assertiveness is a struggle for many of my students. Some come from cultures that emphasize respect for authority, leaving them hesitant to speak up even when it's appropriate. Others have learned that being visible can lead to negative consequences.

I try to create low-stakes situations in which my students can practice advocating for themselves and expressing their thoughts confidently while respecting others.

The final skill in this area is independence. I used to believe I should rely solely on myself. However, I now realize the impor-tance of exercising agency while also knowing when and who to ask for help. Healthy independence involves accountability, considering how actions impact others, and taking responsibility for consequences.

### Interpersonal Skills

These skills include interpersonal relationships, empathy, and social responsibility.

Interpersonal relationships thrive on trust, strong communi-cation, and shared values like integrity. Think of the times when you have invested in a relationship only to find that the other person sees it as transactional or is not willing to put in the work.

Sometimes we want so badly to be liked, accepted, or included that we overlook what is missing.

Healthy relationships require empathy—the ability to acknowledge, understand, and honor others' feelings. However, empathy is only sustainable when we care for our own needs and honor our boundaries. We are not built to be the sole source of emotional support for someone else or to bend until we break.

Finally, social responsibility encourages us to be mindful of how our choices impact the communities we are a part of, from what we consume to acts of kindness or service. This encourages a healthy sense of interdependence, where our actions reflect love for ourselves and others. Consider these words from Fred Rogers: "We live in a world in which we need to share responsibility. It's easy to say, 'It's not my child, not my community, not my world, not my problem.' Then there are those who see the need and respond. I consider those people my heroes."[9]

### Decision-Making

Decision-making encompasses problem-solving, reality testing, and impulse control.

Problem-solving involves managing emotions like discomfort or overwhelm when tackling challenges. Our bodies are wired to seek pleasure. When discomfort arises, it can feel unsafe. This is why procrastination is believed to be driven by emotion. If we associate an upcoming deadline or difficult conversation with negative emotions, we will do everything we can to avoid them. Problem-solving skills allow us to find ways to work through our challenges. Here are some questions you might ask yourself:

What constraints am I facing?
What resources do I have access to?

What have I learned from past experiences that might be
useful?

Where might I need to adapt my plan?

*Reality testing* enables us to move beyond emotions in stressful
situations to see things accurately. It involves discerning which
of our thoughts and beliefs are genuinely rooted in reality. This
process might involve pausing to evaluate our perceptions of a
situation from multiple perspectives before we react. By doing
so, we can identify biases based on our emotions or assumptions
that may be distorting our view of reality.

Another common struggle is *impulse control*—the ability to
avoid risky behavior or shortsighted decisions. Common impulses include reactively lashing out in anger, giving up on goals
prematurely, or distracting yourself through eating or shopping.

When we feel a strong impulse, it can short-circuit our thought
process, making it difficult to see the long-term impact of our
actions clearly. In the moment, trying to resist how we feel often
makes it worse.

One way to get ahead of impulsivity is to brainstorm options
to help us make good decisions, such as meal prep to combat
cravings, wish lists to curb impulse spending, or calling a supportive friend. Also, keep in mind that no one is perfect. We can
move forward from setbacks by accepting reality, reflecting on
what happened, and considering how we might adjust our plan
moving forward.

### Stress Management

Stress management includes *flexibility*, *stress tolerance*, and
*optimism*.

Most of us can agree that life would be a lot less stressful if
everything went just as we planned. However, when we insist that
everything go our way, all our time and energy go into resisting
reality. *Flexibility* encourages us to stay curious, open ourselves

to adjusting our thoughts and feelings as circumstances change, and seek opportunities to learn and grow. It is a helpful tool even in everyday situations when we are struggling to adapt. However, it can be difficult for neurodivergent people such as myself who tend to fall into rigid thinking. We will revisit this in the next mini-retreat.

*Stress tolerance* builds resilience, helping us manage emotions and cope in difficult situations. Over time, we learn to acclimate to common stressors. For instance, when we are babies, we cry when we are hungry but experience less distress as we come to trust that our needs will be met. I have learned to ease myself into unfamiliar situations by finding one thing to focus on—perhaps setting a goal to introduce myself to one person or to learn one thing I did not know before.

The most important tool in my toolkit is *optimism*. At my lowest, the flicker of hope that things might improve kept me going, even if I did not know the details. Optimism isn't about being unrealistic—it's brave to believe in light when you are surrounded by darkness. You don't have to be relentlessly positive; you can still acknowledge reality and experience negative emotions. However, optimism stretches you to consider that the best is possible and helps you to avoid giving up prematurely. It can also be contagious, helping others find the light as well.

I'm usually cool under pressure, but certain triggers rock me to my core. In these moments, I feel like I am eight years old. It helps to take a few deep breaths to assess my needs and identify what is under my control. When I'm able to, I try to find something peaceful or joyful to help shift my emotions. These strategies help me be resilient when life is at its most challenging.

Remember, the aim isn't to avoid stress entirely; some stress is inevitable and can even help motivate us. However, by developing these five components of emotional intelligence, you can strengthen your capacity to tackle challenges and foster resilience.

### Social Intelligence

Now, let's consider how emotional intelligence contributes to social intelligence, helping us to navigate roles and relationships in the world.

Self-awareness of our emotions sets the foundation for improving communication in relationships or workplace performance.

Self-regulation involves taking action to manage our emotions and modify our behavior when they aren't having a desirable impact. Think about a time when you restrained yourself from acting impulsively. Perhaps you knew it wasn't worth damaging a relationship or losing your job. Self-regulation teaches us to have patience with ourselves and others.

Social responsibility reminds us we don't exist solely for ourselves but operate within a greater context, encouraging us to act in ways that positively impact our community.

## REFLECTION

1. Which areas of emotional intelligence do you feel are your strengths? How do you currently practice these in your daily life? Consider how you:
   - Perceive yourself
   - Express yourself
   - Make decisions
   - Navigate interactions with others
   - Cope with stress

2. Where do you see opportunities for growth in your emotional intelligence? In what contexts (e.g., relationships, workplace) might you practice these skills? How could you seek constructive feedback from others to support your growth?

# BUILD AN INTENTIONAL MINDSET

### Fixed and Growth Mindsets

So far, we have learned about our patterns related to our thoughts and emotions, the importance of treating ourselves with compassion, and skills related to emotional intelligence. Now, we are ready to put everything we have learned together to create an intentional mindset.

Think of your mindset as framing your approach to life, helping you to see opportunities for learning and growth even in your obstacles.

Carol Dweck, professor of psychology at Stanford University, has identified two types of mindsets: fixed and growth.[10] A fixed mindset reflects the belief that your abilities and skills are static, while a growth mindset embraces that they can be improved over time.

### Adjusting Your Mindset

I'd like to illustrate how you can transition from a fixed mindset to a growth mindset by sharing three examples from my own life and those I serve. Keep an eye out for some of the cognitive distortions we explored earlier.

The first is the scripted life. It's comfortable, as long as everything goes according to plan. But if something goes awry? Chaos ensues! It's like a game of Jenga—the blocks all come crashing down.

For much of my life, I was overcome by emotions like anger and sadness when things went differently than I anticipated. Shifting to a growth mindset required that I stay open to new possibilities when the unexpected happened, rather than shutting down. By leaning into curiosity, I became more comfortable with asking for help and brainstorming alternatives.

The next example is the belief that to be kind is to be vulnerable. We live in a society that equates kindness with weakness, so we learn instead to be demanding, abrupt, and rigid, insisting on our way. However, a flexible mindset allows us to see everyone around us as individuals with rich backstories. It opens us up to a multitude of possibilities and options.

In the past when I felt stuck, I used to wield my emotions to compel others to act on my behalf. It rarely worked. As I embraced a growth mindset, I found power in compassion and realized that respect and valuing others' time led more often to success. I had uncovered the recipe—embrace reality, adjust, and grow forward.

Lastly, for some of my students, years of having been deprived of opportunities or told what they could not do led to a fixed mindset of learned helplessness. When some of them finally had access to resources, they struggled to leverage them.

In the classroom, I try to create space for them to explore how the fear of failure or believing they are unworthy might hold them back from their dreams. I help them shift how they see themselves and their capabilities by recognizing and validating the fruit of their efforts. If they can learn to embrace curiosity over perfection, take reasonable risks, and ask for help in my classroom, these skills can benefit other aspects of their lives.

I strive to cultivate an environment where growth can thrive—a space where we can all boldly write the next chapter of our stories.

## The Power of a Growth Mindset

Consider mindset work as your opportunity to shift your script for how you see the world and your place in it. Consider it a powerful tool for living with intention, not merely enduring life's storms.

Embracing growth requires you to address the gap between where you are and where you would like to be. As your weaknesses are exposed, you must learn to use mistakes and setbacks as your teachers in order to evolve.

Remember: *Failure is feedback.*

You surrender your need for certainty to move toward what you desire most. In exchange, you hone the ability to conquer your fears.

According to Dweck, a commitment to living with a growth mindset requires ongoing work. In an interview with *The Atlantic*, she states:

> Everyone is a mixture of fixed and growth mindsets. You could have a predominant growth mindset in an area but there can still be things that trigger you into a fixed mindset trait. Something really challenging and outside your comfort zone can trigger it, or, if you encounter someone who is much better than you at something you pride yourself on, you can think "Oh, that person has ability, not me." So I think we all, students and adults, have to look for our fixed-mindset triggers and understand when we are falling into that mindset.[11]

We often believe that if someone is successful in one area of their life, this translates to their capacity in other areas. However, no one is perfect. It is common for us to hide our struggles because we fear that if they were visible, they would contaminate others' impressions of us.

One of the more controversial perspectives regarding mindset is whether we can rely on our own effort, grit, and persistence to crawl out of a fixed mindset and improve our abilities. We cannot.

We live in a society that expects us to pull ourselves up by our bootstraps but does not ensure we all have boots.

Even if hard effort is a large part of one's success, no one is truly self-made. Individual effort is not sufficient.

A growth mindset thrives in an environment of psychological safety—where we feel safe taking risks, making mistakes, and asking for help, trusting that others will not shame us. We benefit from being in community with people who have overcome similar experiences or can go through challenges with us.

When you make a mistake or get stuck, you might feel it's an indicator of your capacity for success. Before you quit, consider that you might be falling into a fixed mindset. To embrace growth, step back to reflect on your approach and explore options for support.

## Moving from a Fixed to a Growth Mindset

Great news: We have already started this work! For example, in chapter 2, we explored affirmations to create a new narrative around our worth, and in chapter 3, we worked on reframing cognitive distortions.

I often get stuck in a fixed mindset when I am doing something that is challenging, and I realize there is no certain roadmap to success. I can lose steam as I get lost in my struggles.

What helps me in this moment is to release perfectionism and take stock of my reality. I try to distinguish which of my thoughts are rooted in truth and which are rooted in fear. I think about what is in my capacity to do at the moment. It is always more reasonable than what I have asked of myself.

I gain a lot of insight from reflecting on my expectations in everyday situations—my insistence on making perfect decisions, wanting to do tasks as quickly as possible, and anticipating how to respond to others before I have fully heard them out.

Are you beginning to sense a pattern here?

It is easy to berate myself for having these tendencies or to compare myself to others—who surely *never* struggle in these ways. However, when I step back, I realize that I can acknowledge how I feel without identifying with it. I am not the sum of my struggles.

From here, I can shift my inner narrative toward a higher level of self-compassion to help my brain relax, which is a game changer. I remind myself that the thoughts I'm having and the resistance I'm feeling are often trying to protect me from failure. They are doing their best to inform me of what I should do based on my previous experiences and beliefs.

Our brains have what is called a negativity bias. They try to protect us from danger by focusing on what could go wrong. They might see the prospect of a minor failure as fatal and avoid it at all costs. You could say that a fixed mindset is a survival technique.

My brain might declare that I should quit now to protect myself. This tendency is often triggered when I am feeling overwhelmed or lack clarity. If I listen, I might give up on something that is important to me. This is an example of when letting go is *not* in our best interest. We cannot afford to surrender our dreams because of a negative prediction in our minds.

We deserve to know how the story plays out.

The good news is, our brains have neuroplasticity, meaning that the way we think is not fixed. We can rewire our brains over time by taking actions that reinforce new patterns of thinking. It takes bravery to speak back to our inner dialogue—especially when it is loud. It is completely normal to have a fixed mindset. But you don't have to stay there.

When I notice that I'm speaking harshly to myself, I might gently reply, "We aren't doing that anymore." I say this to myself as often as needed. It might feel awkward in these moments to offer myself an affirmation, but over time, I begin to believe it.

We can create space between our thoughts and the default reaction of imagining a worst-case scenario by adopting healthier and more effective responses, such as taking time to explore other options or asking for help. Each time we do this, we are programming our brains to respond differently.

We can also rely on the power of community when we feel discouraged about a challenge. I am intentional about reaching out to people who see the best in me but also see me as human. When I am pursuing a new opportunity, I look to connect with people who have relatable experiences or have had success in that area. This helps prevent impostor syndrome, isolation, and doubt from taking root.

It's important to remember that not everything shifts overnight. I still deal with these issues, and as I reach for higher goals, they often intensify.

But even when we lapse, we can *always* return and begin again.

## Process Versus Outcome

One helpful step suggested by Dweck for moving into a growth mindset is to focus on the process rather than the outcome. This allows us to identify the tangible steps that, if taken with consistency, will lead to our end goal. It also gives us the flexibility to adjust along the way. Rather than expecting ourselves to have all the answers, we can become students of the process, ever willing to learn and adapt.

We act by focusing on small steps that represent meaningful progress toward our goal. The trick is to start with something easy so that it is impossible to fail. This helps us to build and sustain momentum, especially when the process is complex.

For example, earning tenure as a professor requires several years of teaching, doing research, writing papers, and engaging in service. It was easy for me to look at this challenge at the beginning and say, "I will never do this." The document listing the requirements was forty-two pages long!

My brain desperately needed to make this feel possible. So, I leaned into one of my strengths: curiosity. I reviewed the document repeatedly, familiarizing myself with its core elements. I simplified them by turning the process into a board game. I set milestones to be achieved and vetted them with my department to ensure they were aligned with their expectations. I tracked details of my progress on a spreadsheet. This simplified the journey for my brain, and ultimately decreased my sense of overwhelm.

Now, I felt safe redirecting my energy from worry to action. I knew that by breaking the process into a series of smaller steps, I only had to follow the sequence to reach my goal.

Suddenly, time spent interacting with students, working on committee projects, or carrying out research were all meaningful parts of the process. I harnessed my ability to hyperfocus by developing a research agenda that was aligned with areas of great interest to me. This motivated me to stay on track. I identified the areas in which I was strong and those I needed help in, then sought out collaborators, mentors, and coaches who could support my growth and success.

Once I had more clarity about my process, I found it easier to turn down requests that were not aligned with or exceeded my capacity. Best of all, when setbacks inevitably happened, I could quickly recover and adapt. This made the process feel much less daunting.

If you have a goal that is worthwhile to you but requires significant time and energy, it is worth taking the time to map out an approach that is both effective and sustainable. When the unexpected unfolds, return to a place of safety and curiosity and identify the smallest possible step forward.

Throughout this chapter we have explored how mindset and emotional intelligence skills can help us manage our thoughts and emotions with intention, informing our behavior. Let's use what we have learned to address the hustle where it shows up in our mental and emotional patterns, identify where to let go, and determine how we can use these skills to cultivate flow and a more intentional mindset.

## Identify the Hustle

When you have a fixed mindset, the hustle can leave you feeling helpless and stuck in overwhelm. This may also involve overthinking, dwelling on worst-case scenarios, masking your needs, or suppressing your emotions. Your actions might look like overreacting to situations, acting impulsively, or letting go prematurely.

Where does the hustle show up most in your thoughts, feelings, and mindset, and how does it affect your actions?

## Cultivate Flow

You can find flow in your life and embrace a growth mindset by reframing cognitive distortions and cultivating your emotional intelligence. This might include using tools or implementing strategies that support your executive function, practicing mindful self-compassion, acknowledging thoughts and feelings neutrally without judgment, engaging in activities that foster positive emotions, finding healthy ways to navigate and express negative emotions, seeking community support, and getting help with mental health challenges.

How can you introduce sustainable practices to positively impact your mental health moving forward?

## Know Where to Let Go

As you move from a fixed to a growth mindset, examples of what to let go of might include unrealistic expectations of never experiencing negative emotions, limiting beliefs, learned helplessness, and distorted thinking patterns.

Those of us who've experienced anxiety know it's not as simple as deciding to let go of thoughts or stop overthinking. Similarly, depression and other mood disorders can intensify our experience of negative emotions and hinder our ability to feel positive ones. For example, I'll likely continue to navigate challenges related to my AuDHD (Autism and ADHD)—that's not something I can let go of.

What can you and might you want to let go of? What *is* within your control to release to address distorted thinking, enhance your emotional intelligence, or ground your thoughts in reality? Where might you benefit from support? Consider asking someone you trust to share their insights on what might help you move forward.

## REFLECTION

1. **Mindset and upbringing:** Growing up, were you encouraged to have a fixed or growth mindset? How were these mindsets modeled by those around you, and how did that impact your own approach?
2. **Fixed mindset:** Describe a time you had a fixed mindset and felt you couldn't overcome a challenge. What beliefs were holding you back?
3. **From fixed to growth:** Recall a specific instance when you shifted from a fixed to a growth mindset. What strategies, such as engaging in learning or curiosity, helped you make this change? What support did you receive, and how did this impact your approach to challenges?

### An Inclusive Approach to Wellness

Earlier in the chapter, we spoke about cognitive flexibility—the ability to think about multiple concepts at once or shift our behavior in response to changes in our environment. It helps us be creative and resilient, solve problems, and navigate uncertainty.

One feature of my Autism is monotropism—the tendency to focus intensely on a small number of things to the exclusion of other things going on around me. This negatively impacts my cognitive function because I struggle to manage my attention and may neglect other important tasks. I have learned that while I do benefit from time to pursue special interests, I also need supportive techniques to help me understand the importance of other tasks and shift my attention to them. I may ask lots of questions or rehearse in my mind how I will approach a situation. All of this helps me feel more confident about moving beyond my comfort zone.

We can build cognitive flexibility by

- trying new things,
- challenging ourselves gradually,
- exploring ways to modify our typical routines, and
- meeting people who broaden our perspective.

Cognitive flexibility helped me overcome a great barrier in my mental health journey—resistance to medication. I had to acknowledge past experiences I'd had with medications that had left me feeling numb, groggy, or experiencing severe side effects. I also struggled with internalized ableism around the idea of being a wellness expert who needed more than retreats or meditation to be well.

For a long time, I held out hope that I could find the right set of strategies that would eliminate this need (internalized ableism dies hard). However, my intensifying struggles with anxiety and depression finally led me to reconsider. I needed the support of a patient and well-informed health care team dedicated to finding solutions that work for me. Although it is an ongoing journey, I have found the combination of medication and effective tools, systems, and strategies to be beneficial for my personal journey.

Therapy has also been a wonderful resource in helping me understand and process my experiences. In the past, I have frequently been graduated from therapy by professionals who believed that my positive outlook and ability to achieve at a high level meant that I had the tools I needed to cope. I now know that it may be hard for others to see when I am suffering, so having a therapist who can see beyond my mask and understand my journey with AuDHD is essential.

I honor that we all have unique needs and preferences when it comes to treatments such as therapy and medication. However, I find it important to acknowledge broader societal factors, such as cultural stigma and barriers to access, affordability, and receiving culturally relevant care from empathetic practitioners.

In many cultures with a history of marginalization, like the Black community, there's a deep mistrust of health care systems that have treated them poorly, deprived them of access to quality services, and subjected them to experimentation and sterilization without consent, to name a few examples. Mistrust is reinforced today by ongoing negative experiences with providers and systems, including the perpetuation of negative stereotypes and false beliefs, such as the falsehood that Black people have thicker skin and thus have a higher threshold for pain.

Many health disparities are rooted in inequity. Issues like safe housing, access to food, employment, and freedom from discrimination are the drivers of many mental health challenges in marginalized communities. Being vulnerable can come at a risk if it results in being labeled by the system and subjected to ongoing discrimination. Harmful behaviors such as substance misuse must be seen in context. While not absolving accountability, it is important to acknowledge that people may be attempting to cope with their struggles using the resources they have access to.

Restoring trust requires not just acknowledging harm but taking steps to address systemic issues that perpetuate it. This includes providing equitable care and addressing concerns about the safety and effectiveness of medication by improving the representation of marginalized communities in research. To foster trust, there must be a commitment to inviting those who have been harmed to the table to determine the path forward.

Once practitioners have been trained on trauma- and shame-informed practices, they can create spaces in which patients may feel safer being open and vulnerable about their experiences. A mindset of cultural humility encourages providers to address their biases and ensures that the patient's perspective of their experience and their desires regarding treatment are both solicited and honored. Practitioners can invite patients to share aspects of their identity and lived experiences, such as cultural beliefs and traditional practices, to be considered in their care plan.

Finally, we need to raise awareness of the diverse therapeutic approaches available. It was only after a decade of talk therapy that I discovered somatic practices that are helpful in reprocessing traumatic memories, such as EMDR, ART, somatic experiencing, and brainspotting.*

However, it was a comedy sketch that ultimately spurred me to action. In her HBO comedy special, *Momma, I Made It!*, Yvonne Orji—known for her role on HBO's *Insecure*—praised EMDR for helping her navigate life's challenges. Her relatable story convinced me that if it worked for her, it might work for me too. Somatic practices equipped me with tools to better regulate my emotions, which meant I was no longer suppressing them.

Looking back at my own introduction to meditation, I struggled for years to find a practice that worked for me. I would have benefited from culturally tailored practices that considered my needs as a Black neurodivergent woman. Through trial and error, I realized the strategies that I was being taught needed to be adapted for my own reality.

Meditation works best in my life as a daily mental reset. It is a brief period of time when I can pause what I am doing to allow myself to just be present and observe how I feel. If I have thoughts the entire time, no problem. I call it "taking the trash out." My aim is to show up for myself without agenda or expectation.

---

*EMDR stands for eye movement desensitization and reprocessing; ART stands for accelerated resolution therapy.

In return, meditation provides a space for me to breathe and disconnect from my thoughts and the world. I envision that I am on the surface of the ocean, and as I meditate, I begin to sink deeper and deeper.

I came up with this visualization after a scuba diving experience. I felt so calm when the only noises I could hear were of the water, and the only job I had was to breathe and be present. When I meditate, I allow the emotions that are weighing me down to decrease in intensity and sometimes even float away. Afterward, I often feel energized and able to return to my day with a renewed focus and perspective.

Through embracing a growth mindset, I will continue to find new ways to support my needs as I evolve. I may have a different approach a year from now, as I will be on a new leg of my journey. But for now, my intentions are to embrace presence rather than perfection, and to learn to savor and appreciate where I am today.

For all of us, therapy and medical treatment should be paired with individual and community approaches to care for our mental health. Individuals can incorporate practices such as meditation or journaling as a way to process thoughts and emotions, but this processing can also happen in a group of trusted friends or people who have gone through similar experiences. Support groups and activities such as sound healing can facilitate healing in community, helping us to coregulate. We can engage in healing as a collective, learning new ways to manage our stress and emotions from others, strengthening the bonds of our common humanity in the process.

# 5

# Flaws and All

*Your Body's Journey*

I once shaved off half an eyebrow using a razor, trying to fit in.

I have always felt connected to my body in some ways and disconnected in others. I love to sing and dance and was taught from a young age to embrace my honey-caramel skin. However, when I entered junior high, I started to view my body through the lens of my peers. It was no longer whole, but a series of parts to be judged and measured individually for their worth.

They carefully studied my forehead, my nose, my stomach—all deemed too big. I took note of my weight, as if it were an indicator of my value, a problem to be solved. I looked at photos and saw how my broad shoulders stood out, no matter how hard I tried to blend in. No matter how I tried to have a sense of style, it was hopeless. I gave up, convincing myself I did not care.

I was only interested in what my body could *do* for me. I needed it to carry me to my destination, hold emotions I was uncomfortable expressing, and most of all, fit in.

So I ignored its signals. I was resentful of pain, rarely treating it until it became unbearable. When my feelings became overwhelming, I learned how to soothe them with food. I did not know how to have a reciprocal relationship with my body, to show it praise for its generous gifts of breath and heartbeats. I rarely noticed—let alone acknowledged—its efforts.

I had no way of knowing that tuning out the bad also meant tuning out the good.

I missed out on years of appreciating that what I had was more than enough. To me, my mind was the prize. It was the vessel that could take me places—the tool that would help me achieve success beyond my wildest dreams.

In contrast, my body felt like an inconvenience, a reminder of my flaws, something to be controlled. Having grown up in the wake of the AIDS epidemic and the advent of purity culture, disconnecting from my body became a strategy for success—the ultimate chess move.

No one told me how to plug back in.

I learned through trial and error. Leaning into diets and fitness regimens that—no matter how successful—never left me feeling better about myself. I couldn't see beyond the number on the scale.

The process of building trust with my body took time. I had to unravel all the narratives that kept me at a distance from myself. My body had so much to say to me—it was just waiting for me to listen without judgment. As I became more fluent in its language, I learned its likes and dislikes, which sensations signaled joy, hope, or excitement, and which indicated discomfort.

I have learned that my body is never as upset at me as I have been with it. It waited for me to accept what it knew all along— that I was not designed to fit in but to stand out. With every breath, I am reminded of its love and dedication. With every step I take to fully embrace life, I love it back.

Loving ourselves is a vital daily practice that helps us find our way back home.

## The Beauty in Our Flaws

For years, I have been drawn to *kintsugi*, a Japanese art form used to restore broken pottery and other objects. *Kintsugi* translates to "gold joinery." This art form involves reconnecting broken pieces using lacquer and a delicate powder of gold or other precious metals.

The cracks, which tell a story of brokenness, are filled with gold, transforming them into elegant lines that elevate the object's value. This is a restorative process that celebrates renewal, highlighting imperfections as part of the larger story rather than concealing them.

*Kintsugi* aligns with the Japanese philosophy of *wabi-sabi*: embracing beauty and simplicity amid life's impermanence and imperfection. It teaches us that while we can't control what happens to us, we can control our response, creating new narratives as we embrace the healing process.

The vessel in *kintsugi* represents our human experience. We endure pressure from difficult life experiences that can break us in unpredictable ways.

Our wellness journey—using gold to fill the cracks—starts with self-acceptance. Through this process, we restore connection and affirm our wholeness. We come to see our imperfections, even those we continue to struggle with, as part of our unique narrative of what it means to live in this body. We embrace the transient nature of life by choosing to be present, living beyond what has transpired.

Some wounds can be repaired with love, time, and other resources, but the memories linger. Other losses are irreparable. We repair what we can, learn when to let go, and find a way to appreciate what remains. These experiences challenge us to transform and grow—building resilience as we shed what we can no longer carry.

Reflecting on our bodies' stories allows us to see our perseverance, broadening our capacity for healing and growth. Let's explore together our relationships with our bodies and how we can care for them.

## RETREAT RESET

Take a moment to connect with your body.

Introduce some small movements to help anchor yourself where you are. For example, you can wiggle your fingers and toes, rotate your head slowly in both directions, and shrug your shoulders up and down. You can ground yourself by visualizing your bottom anchored into your chair or feet anchored into the ground.

Imagine there are roots extending deep into the earth, providing you with stability and support. If you are feeling stressed, try to make your exhale twice as long as your inhale. This may help activate your body's relaxation response.

While I encourage you to review the safety check included after the book's introduction (see page 27) at any point while reading this book, I want to specifically encourage you to do this in preparation for this chapter's sections. If you choose to review that, do so now.

Grounding exercises can help you reestablish connection with yourself when you are experiencing difficult emotions. Here are two examples of activities you might find helpful. Take a moment to try them out and reflect on your experience.

### Body Scan

1. Start with several slow, deep breaths.
2. Focus on sensations in your feet or head.
3. Move your attention up or down, to one body part at a time.
4. Reverse direction, returning to the original body part.

*Sensory Scavenger Hunt*

1. Name five things that you can see.
2. Name four things that you can touch.
3. Name three things that you can hear.
4. Name two things that you can smell.
5. Name one thing that you can taste.

As you return to this moment, what were you aware of in your body? How do you feel right now?

When you are ready, let's continue this journey together.

MINI-RETREAT #1:

# YOUR BODY IS WORTHY . . . PERIOD

## Restoring Connection with Your Body

Our relationships with our bodies are complex, partly because they are always evolving and changing. If you idealize one version of yourself, you might struggle with changes such as aging or weight gain.

Practices to foster body compassion can help you develop more compassion toward your body and a healthy body image. Body compassion has three parts:[1]

1. Defusion: The extent to which your attitude about your body leads to isolating from others, judging yourself, or over-identifying with your flaws
2. Common humanity: Reminding yourself that you are not alone, that others have similar experiences and feelings regarding their own bodies
3. Acceptance: Accepting all aspects of your body, including how you feel, your appearance, and your flaws

The aim is to decrease defusion and increase common humanity and acceptance. It is important to note that these practices take time, and you may require support. Forcing yourself to feel something that you do not might only serve to increase the resistance and disconnection that you feel.

Body neutrality may be another helpful pathway to restoring connection to and care for yourself. This way of thinking focuses on what your body can *do* rather than just what it *looks* like. And you can focus on honoring your body for what it is able to do today without making a moral judgment.

Remember, no matter how you feel, your body is still enough. Because it exists.

Your body is the vessel for your mind and spirit that makes it possible to experience life and be present with those you love.

Your body is not the barometer for your worth. Physical care is not a practice of perfecting your body but of using the resources you have to nourish your body and preserve your ability to function in daily life.

## Restoring Connection

Using body compassion or body neutrality as our starting point, we can work toward restoring (or perhaps building for the first time) real connection with our bodies.

During a wellness retreat I was conducting for higher education staff, I went through a series of exercises (such as the body scan featured in the retreat reset at the beginning of this chapter) to help participants connect with the sensations in their bodies. A Black woman in the audience shared that it was the first time she had ever intentionally thought about being present in her body.

I can relate. I have always found it easier to pay attention to my thoughts and projects I am working on than to the signals being sent by my body for nourishment, movement, or a break. I experience sensory challenges that make it harder to hear and honor my body's needs. Even when I sense that I am hungry, thirsty, tired, or need to go to the restroom, it's a quiet whisper compared to my reluctance to break my focus. I push a few minutes more, and a few minutes more . . . until it is impossible to ignore.

For years, I prided myself on being able to push through boredom, exhaustion, and discomfort to get work done. I ignored warning signs such as eye strain or shoulder pain that told me I needed to take breaks.

These habits were reinforced by my environment in academia, where many of us embrace a "work hard, play hard" mentality. Tiredness is fixed by caffeine or sugar (until the next crash!). The ability to sit and read for hours is an asset. I learned to work through exhaustion until it gave way to a second wind that would allow me to complete my task. Over time, I found it difficult to stop—even when I wanted to.

The result was increased chronic pain.

I don't fault myself or anyone else who feels disconnected from their body; this takes time and consistent attention to unravel. Starting in kindergarten, we go from moving freely to being taught to stay in our seats until we are told otherwise. As we progress in our education, we learn to study late into the night. In adulthood, many of our roles encourage us to be sedentary.

Stress also affects physical wellness in many ways. Pain is a signal from our nervous system that everything isn't all right. When our stress response system is activated repeatedly, changes like increased inflammation are early warning signs that, if ignored, become risk factors for disease.

It doesn't have to be this way.

Many of the conditions that are prevalent in our society are preventable or treatable if we pay attention to the signs our bodies send and take appropriate action.

The way we restore connection to our bodies is by *listening* to them, honoring and addressing their needs for nourishment and rest.

You can nurture an ongoing conversation with your body by practicing awareness. Note your feelings and your inner dialogue. Pay attention to your behavioral patterns and how they impact your body. Think about the following:

1. What do you want your body to be able to do as you navigate this world?
2. How do you want it to feel?

Remember, your body and its needs will evolve throughout your life. It's relying on you to show up for it where it is today.

### Honoring the Whole Body

Caring for yourself (mind, body, and spirit) requires you to honor your body and all it has endured. My body is a reminder of all I have survived, from scars left by health events to scrapes that are the souvenirs of adventures to the reminder that my hand is not a great cat toy.

Our bodies show up for us every day of our lives, from supporting our ability to engage in daily activities to experiencing the thrill of a new challenge and providing a warm embrace to a loved one. We cannot outsource the work of our bodies to others.

How can we care for our bodies in return?

A holistic approach to wellness starts with the ability to nurture our bodies, free from shame that comes from ourselves and others. We can honor our bodies by

- practicing being present in this moment,
- wearing clothes that fit and honor the bodies we have today,
- letting go of an ideal shape or level of athletic skill, and
- not judging the changes or enhancements that we or others make to our bodies.

These acts of care can help us to heal from past shame, sending the message that our bodies are worthy. In turn, we strengthen the capacity of our bodies to show up for us as we navigate life.

### Releasing Judgment

As you reflect on these words, you may be reminded of some of the judgment you have experienced from others.

When other people judge you, they are often projecting their own fears or standards onto you or acting out of a misguided desire to protect you. Perhaps someone has told you that you are too sensitive and need to be stronger—and that comments like those are "supposed to toughen you up."

No matter how well-intentioned they consider themselves to be, these comments do significant damage when they come from the ones who claim to love us unconditionally. They reinforce a narrative that we must change ourselves to be worthy of acceptance or love.

What they say about your body is not the truth about you.

You are worthy simply because *you exist*. And no one can take that from you.

In the following sections, we will explore how to care for ourselves with compassion and grace, honoring our authentic needs rather than administering shame—which only drives us farther from ourselves and each other.

## REFLECTION

Take a moment to reflect on your relationship with your body. You may choose any format that resonates with you, such as a letter, poem, drawing, or vision board. Below is a poem I wrote about my own experiences.

### Acceptance

I feel good about my body
(Mostly)

Except for those moments,
Typically in the morning, when I linger in the mirror
(And sometimes on the scale)
And request a leaner version of myself.
As if I could order her in the mirror.
As if she could become me. Instantly.

Except for those moments
Any other time of the day
Standing or sitting down
When I catch a glance of my midsection
And fall out of love with myself.

This self that conducts my breath
Drums my heartbeat
Fuels my dreams
We disconnect and drift apart.

The repair is lengthy, costly.
Sometimes I forget my way back

As someone else's narrative
Of how to exist in my own body
Gets trapped inside.

Eventually, I discern the difference between
This foreign voice and me
Who is proud of this body
The scars that hold witness
Of all it has overcome.

As I take one step back toward myself
I choose clothing as a way to celebrate
Rather than hide the body I have today
I add earrings, glasses, and lip gloss
A peace offering.

We make up.
And once again, silence the narrative
That tells me I am not enough.

We will do this again and again
As often as necessary
Knowing this practice
This dance
Of always returning
Is love.

MINI-RETREAT #2:

## CARE FOR YOUR BODY'S UNIQUE NEEDS

### How to Care for the Body You Have Now

I've noticed a common pattern among many of my clients who want to focus on their physical activity. Many can recall a time when they were more active, before long work hours and desk jobs took over. It's not enough for them to start where they are now; they expect their bodies to perform on par with their peak physical condition. This mindset often prevents them from starting at all.

I can relate to how they feel. By reflecting on my own peak experiences, I have learned to reframe my concept of my personal best.

In grad school, I trained to run a marathon with my father, who had taken up running a decade prior. We trained on the beach in Santa Monica and in the hills of Pacific Palisades, so motivation for shorter distances came easily.

However, the day we set out for fourteen miles, I had to rethink my commitment. About halfway through, I felt I couldn't go on. I quickly learned that this was a common experience referred to as "hitting the wall." The wall is different for everyone. It represents the farthest you believe you can go. In that moment, your body starts pleading for you to stop, convincing you that you have nothing more to give. The point is to push through to the other side, to see what you are made of.

At that moment, I wanted to be made of a nap, but I was far from my car, so I continued.

Gradually, my strength and confidence returned, and I realized I was capable of more than I'd given myself credit for. When I ran the full marathon later that year, I hit my wall around mile seventeen, and the feeling stuck with me through mile twenty. I didn't want to talk to anybody; I just wanted the race to be over.

However, this time I knew I didn't have to give up because there would be a surge of energy on the other side. Sure enough, while miles twenty-one through twenty-six were still unfathomably long, they felt more doable.

I am so grateful to have experienced these highs. I had no idea that the health events I described at the beginning of this book would take place one year later.

It has been a humbling process to learn how to honor my capacity.

My personal best now is where I show up for myself today. It is everything I do to care for myself with the resources and constraints I have. I hit the wall whenever I am overwhelmed by a new health challenge. I have been here so many times that it has become familiar. Each time, I pause to regain my footing.

Then, I focus on taking the next step.

## Developing Your Care Plan

In this mini-retreat, you will engage in self-awareness to identify your authentic needs related to nourishment, movement, and sleep.

Engaging in this practice with compassion for yourself will allow you to discover *your* personal best for your current reality.

### Nourishment

Nourishing your body is not about finding the perfect diet but about fueling your body with nutrients so that you have the energy you need to engage in daily life. This includes finding sustainable ways to meet your body's nutritional needs and ensuring that you are hydrating regularly.

What works for you may be different from what works for others around you. For example, I struggle with meal prep. I felt shame about this for some time because I used to love cooking and was good at it. Suddenly, I found it very hard to follow recipes.

I had to pivot. Through trial and error, I identified a core menu I'm willing to choose from for each meal. This menu is made up of foods that are aligned with my nutritional needs but require little to no preparation. This realistic approach reduces decision fatigue and makes it easier to feed myself when I am short on time or energy.

### Movement

You rely on your body to show up for you in every aspect of your life. Engaging in regular movement promotes your cardiovascular health and helps reduce stress, while preserving your body's functionality and strength. It is important to find practices that are beneficial for you and appropriate for your ability and level of skill.

If you find activities that are meaningful or enjoyable for you and can be integrated into your daily life, you are more likely to be consistent.

Movement looks different for each of us, reflecting our needs, preferences, and abilities. Focus on what is realistic for you. While I no longer run marathons, I enjoy walking, cycling, dancing, yoga, and other activities. I have learned not to push myself beyond my limits. This requires paying attention to my level of exertion and taking immediate action if I experience pain. I have let go of one-size-fits-all approaches to fitness and instead work with people who have specialized training to support my needs.

### Sleep

While we all know that sleep is crucial for our health, many of us struggle to get enough rest. Those with intense work schedules, young children, or other caregiving responsibilities often find sleep elusive. Others grapple with insomnia for any number of reasons. Sleep is an important aspect of our health, but it is one where we all need to extend grace to ourselves based on our reality.

I spent years struggling with sleep, mostly obsessing over how little of it I was getting. It took about a decade of exploring options with various medical teams before my AuDHD diagnosis finally gave context to my struggles. Even with medication to support me, I know that some days I might be too overstimulated to fall asleep or might wake up early. I try to accept my reality and not strive for perfection. Some days I recover well, and on others, I have to adjust my expectations.

If I've learned anything concrete, it's that your best strategies are probably not my best strategies, and vice versa. Our experiences related to sleep are as unique as we are. Rather than feeling guilty about poor sleep habits, approach your experience with curiosity. Consider the factors affecting your sleep and explore supportive practices that are sustainable for you.

## REFLECTION

Reflect on your past patterns and current practices related to nourishment, movement, and sleep.

1. Which of them have contributed to hustle, in that they are unsustainable or unrealistic for you or based on harmful expectations and assumptions?
2. What can you let go of? What is not under your control to let go of (i.e., it's part of your reality or is an ongoing challenge)?
3. How can you cultivate flow? Identify practices that are sustainable and will support your overall well-being in daily life.

## MINI-RETREAT #3:
# BECOME THE CAPTAIN OF YOUR HEALTH CARE TEAM

### Maintaining Your Body Through Preventive Care

The cornerstone of my field, public health, is preventive care. However, this is not easy. It can take significant time, energy, and financial resources to schedule annual physicals, obtain recommended screenings based on your age and risk factors, and follow through with treatment regimens for medication, physical therapy, and other procedures.

While caring for your body's needs can be inconvenient, the alternative of dealing with preventable injuries and illnesses is far worse. So, it's important to start simple. Spend time observing your physical appearance and the sensations you feel so that you are more likely to notice changes.

Take action when you first detect signs of pain or something abnormal. I could have saved hundreds of hours in physical therapy if I'd stopped before pushing myself beyond my limits, or thought twice about carrying a forty-liter backpack for several weeks throughout Asia.

It's impossible to prevent everything. You don't have to know all the answers, but it's up to you to advocate for yourself by asking questions. My kidney disease diagnosis was the result of deciding to visit my doctor because something didn't feel right. Although it took months to detect what was wrong, from there we took swift action to stop the damage and promote my quality of life. I am grateful every day that I listened to that feeling and spoke up.

Honoring your body means caring for it throughout the course of your life. It may feel overwhelming at times, but allowing issues to pile up leads to greater consequences. Do what you can to be diligent about staying on top of the steps needed for your ongoing care and recovery.

## Complex Health Issues

Prioritizing your care becomes more complicated when dealing with complex health issues, as it's even more important to be an advocate for your own health.

*You* are the expert on your body and experiences. Honor your limits and needs, especially those that may be dismissed by others.

It can be isolating to navigate chronic illness, cancer, or other complex health issues. It is important not to do it alone. My life changed drastically, as I suddenly had different priorities (and very little energy). I was incredibly grateful to have the support of my mother, who went out to find me work clothes after I had rapidly gained twenty pounds in just a few months.

However, few of my friends could relate to the challenges I was going through. I drew very close to the ones who did. We could go from expressing sadness about our latest lab results or frustration over our pain and low energy to humorous exchanges about the ridiculous nature of our predicaments. I also embraced online spaces where I could find others with similar experiences.

My greatest motivation for caring for my complex health needs is to avoid burnout. In the context of chronic illness, this looks like being so overwhelmed by the ongoing stress of managing your condition that you lose the motivation or the ability to keep up with your care.*

Ongoing experiences of physical and mental pain can be depleting, especially when you have to navigate a world that is not

---

*There are some specific types of burnout that are being increasingly discussed, such as burnout related to Autism or ADHD, which might leave someone incapacitated to the point that they cannot work for months or years, if ever again. We will discuss burnout in other contexts in chapter 7.

set up to be compassionate or responsive to your needs. Others may not understand and may feel that you are making excuses, especially if your condition is permanent, prolonged, not easily resolved, invisible, or requires support that is perceived to be inconvenient.

In my own experience, I've come to accept that medicine is far more of an art than a science. Some of my symptoms went for years without being correctly diagnosed, and I experienced a fair amount of unsupportive treatment from providers who saw my questions and cautions as inconvenient and unhelpful.

I had to renegotiate my relationship with my body with each new diagnosis or unexpected health event.

Over time, I learned to notice when I was tackling too many health issues at once. Sometimes I felt like a detective, chasing clues to get to the bottom of my most recent diagnosis. Other times, I felt like an executive assistant trying to navigate appointment schedules for multiple providers along with the responsibilities of my personal and professional life.

But mostly, I feel like a professional patient.

Doing my best on any particular day starts with taking the most basic steps to manage my condition, such as measuring my blood pressure and taking my medications. This consistency pays off over time.

I get tears in my eyes when I think about the positive feedback I have received from my providers recently. One commented on my improved energy now that I have been sleeping more. Another thanked me for the effort I put into creating monthly health updates that compile everyone's recommendations along with my own observations. My therapist congratulated me for all the work I have done to build my self-worth, maintain boundaries, and improve my mental health.

We have so many things to address, but these moments remind me to pause and celebrate how far I've come, and to be grateful for everything that is going well.

I can't believe all that I have had to go through to protect my wellness. It has stretched me far beyond what I thought I was capable of. So, while society might try to pick out all my imperfections, it means everything to me to know that my providers who actually know the depth of my struggles are cheering on my progress.

Celebrate any and all wins available to you. This journey can be very unaccommodating, from navigating the health care system to juggling the management of your condition with parenting, work, and other responsibilities.

Few of us have time to be professional patients. But we can be our own best advocates, focusing on what *we can* control and using the resources we have access to in order to make informed decisions about our health.

## REFLECTION

1. What health care needs are a priority for you to address right now?
2. Consider a time when you have felt resistant to caring for yourself. What do you think you needed in that moment?
3. What have you learned from your previous experiences that can help you care for your needs moving forward?

MINI-RETREAT #4:

# FIND THE RIGHT FLOW FOR YOUR BODY

### Uncovering How Hustle Culture Impacts Your Body

Although there is increasingly diverse representation of body sizes and types, the body image most often considered to be ideal is youthful, flawless . . . and inaccessible to most of us who lack a specific genetic predisposition or the resources to achieve and maintain these beauty standards.

We learn to ignore pain, thirst, hunger, and exhaustion in pursuit of productivity, ultimately at the expense of our well-being.

This mindset keeps us perpetually at odds with our bodies. In our quest for "optimal health" and endless youth, we often deplete our resources and become even more disconnected from our body's authentic needs.

The myth of the perfect body leaves no room for imperfection, injury, or illness.

We are consistently fed unrealistic expectations that make it challenging to cope with reality. Furthermore, access to quality health care often depends on financial resources. The communities we live in significantly influence the quality of care we receive, our available resources, and even our life expectancy. Nonetheless, the responsibility for health is often placed on the individual.

We were not made to be at constant odds with our bodies. It doesn't have to be this way. Let's take stock together of where we are in our current reality, name our hustle, figure out where to let go, and learn how to cultivate our own flow.

**Identify the Hustle**

The hustle has shown up for me in several of the practices discussed in this chapter.

As explored in my poem, my relationship with my body is a complex dance. I often struggle with expectations I have internalized from society and my culture about what my body should look like. I've spent a lot of time and energy trying to find the perfect diet. This is absolutely informed by diet culture, which has never failed to produce a new fad to capture my attention, promising to address all my pain points.

The greater the promise, the harder the fall.

The hustle shows up for me when I try to push myself to extremes, signaling that I am not operating from a place of connection with my body. It happens when

- I withhold the variety of nutrients that help me feel nourished,
- I avoid gathering in community or making social plans that involve food, or
- I push myself beyond my limits in workouts, my professional roles, or showing up for others because I am not conscious of my energy limits.

If we feel negatively about our bodies, it's important to recognize that these feelings are learned, often from unrealistic ideals of perfection. And when we develop the awareness to identify where feelings of resistance toward ourselves stem from and what triggers them, we can better address our needs.

## Know Where to Let Go

We must let go of other people's standards, societal standards, and our own unrealistic standards that don't honor what we've been through or need.

I have had to dismiss the narrative that I should push through pain and cover up flaws because only perfect bodies deserve to be loved and nourished.

In terms of nourishment, letting go of diet culture and embracing body compassion is an ongoing journey. There are still some remnants of diet culture in the back of my mind that are triggered by certain practices or the promises offered by the latest trend.

In regard to movement, I have learned to move in sync with the needs of my body. With the support of a trainer, I set realistic goals for strength and cardiovascular training that are effective and sustainable, increasing my stability and overall function without risking injury.

## Cultivate Flow

Finding the right flow for your body is about identifying the approach that works best for you. Here are some things I've learned as I've cultivated my own body's flow.

### What Makes Me Feel Good

I've learned that my relationship with my body improves when I pay attention to what makes me feel good, from the clothing I wear to the pace I move through life at.

### What Relieves Stress

Over time, I have had to learn how stress shows up in my body and how I can address it. I wear a nightguard at night to protect my teeth from grinding in my sleep. Activities like walking, stretching, and yoga help release tension in my neck, shoulders, and back. Therapies like EMDR have helped my body find relief as it processes stored emotions.

### What Keeps Me Present in My Body

I have learned many tools to help myself stay present in my body and restore connection when it has been disrupted. Because my body's signals are not always easy for me to detect or honor, alarms and schedules can help remind me to eat, hydrate, and take breaks for movement or going outside.

Do I do this perfectly? Absolutely not. I mess it up all the time. However, my goal is to be a student of my own process, reflecting on where my systems fall short. This will help me better discern what works best for me.

## What Sustains Me

Nourishment and movement are two areas where I have worked hard to establish flow. I have learned to be flexible with my plans based on my capacity to ensure I meet my end goal. For example, when it comes to nutrition, the most important thing is to ensure I have food available, whether that involves ordering groceries, making simpler meals, or choosing prepared options.

For movement, my aim is to build and maintain the functional strength I need to engage in daily life and age well. Over time, I have found that the most sustainable approach for me involves gentle, consistent movement.

This allows me to select from a range of activities that will progress me toward my goals while honoring my limits. It acknowledges that there will be days I don't engage in movement at all. That's reality. Consistency is not about perfection but a commitment to resume the process from wherever I am. While it has taken time to develop this approach, it has paid off in building a trusting relationship with my body.

## REFLECTION

1. Where does the hustle show up in your life, making it more difficult for you to care for your physical needs or other areas of wellness?

2. What are you holding on to that you can release in order to care for yourself in a more sustainable manner? Consider societal standards or expectations you may have internalized from the projections of others that are not realistic for or aligned with your values.

3. What is not under your control to release, or would take significant time and effort to do so?

4. Which of your existing practices are sustainable, realistic, and desirable for you? What practices do you think would

be desirable for you to incorporate into your daily life to cultivate flow?

## An Inclusive Approach to Wellness

We must acknowledge systemic barriers to wellness, such as racism and discrimination in the health care system. People shouldn't be treated differently based on their sexual orientation, immigration status, gender, or ethnicity—but they are.

Many people do not have the luxury to prioritize their health amid their responsibilities or limited access to resources. Marginalized communities often delay care due to lack of access, stigma, and mistrust.[2] This delay in screening can lead to later diagnoses, making it harder to treat conditions that may have been preventable or treatable if identified earlier through screenings and annual checkups.

In a study I coauthored on Black women receiving care at a safety net hospital in Alabama, participants who reported experiences of discrimination based on race, gender, or race *and* gender were more likely to report lower mental well-being and had lower rates of physician trust.[3]

I've personally encountered doctors who made assumptions about me, were insensitive to my needs, or made me feel bad for my situation, as if it were fully under my control. Others became defensive when I asked questions regarding my condition or care. While I value and seek out their expertise, *I* have to live out the consequences of any actions we take. If I let these interactions discourage me from addressing my needs, who will advocate for me?

After I was diagnosed with kidney disease, I extensively researched it and learned about potential complications, including an increased risk of blood clots. At the same time, I was experiencing extreme pain during my menstrual cycles.

I was prescribed a medication that also had a side effect of increased risk of blood clots. I expressed my concern to my ob-gyn, but he dismissed my concerns, saying I would be fine. I knew it was important but ultimately prioritized addressing the pain.

I ended up having a blood clot three months later.

When I look back at the times I was led to second-guess myself or feel bad for being human, I know I don't want that for anybody else. We need to do better.

These experiences have helped me clarify what I am looking for when it comes to selecting a provider. I want someone who is skilled, curious, collaborative, and compassionate. I have to feel safe enough with my provider to be open and honest about my experiences and concerns. While there is no guarantee you will find an ideal match, I encourage you to think about the qualities that are important to you and keep them in mind when meeting with providers.

You deserve compassionate care, no matter your circumstances or health needs.

If you feel disrespected or that your needs are being overlooked, honor your instincts and speak up so that you may receive the best care possible. I realize I may be challenging you to navigate a system that likely wasn't built for you, but I want you to use the tools and resources you have access to in order to make informed decisions.

For example, many of us have a hard time talking about end-of-life care and advance directives. Many doctors hesitate to bring up the conversation because of the discomfort they anticipate. However, none of us know when we might need to have this in place. While we often focus on older generations for these discussions, if you want your family to address these issues, the best thing you can do is to start learning about them for yourself. You may end up inspiring someone else in your circle to do the same. And when they need a resource, you will be prepared.

I'm grateful that I educated myself on these topics and taught on them in my classes. I was prepared when I had to sign my own paperwork before a major surgery. Later, when my family needed to make difficult decisions for another member, I was able to step up and provide helpful information. I want you to have that option, too, so you can feel more empowered to support your loved ones and address your own needs.

Finally, consider options for medical care beyond Western medicine you may have access to. For example, *integrative medicine* includes not only standard medical care but also complementary and alternative medicine (e.g., traditional remedies and healing practices, acupuncture, yoga, massage, somatic experiencing).

When it comes to your health care needs, the ultimate authority rests with *you*. Explore practices to find what is right for your unique body.

# 6

# Support Squad

## The Importance of Community
## in a Complex World

I am what Malcolm Gladwell referred to as a connector in his book *The Tipping Point*.

I enjoy meeting people in different worlds, learning what motivates them, understanding their needs, and connecting them with the resources or support they need to move forward. I prefer deep, rich conversations over surface-level connections. And if there are one hundred people in a room, I'd rather be outside on the patio, getting to know two or three of them and enjoying fresh air.

Quality over quantity.

Up until a few years ago, I would have spoken to everyone in the room. I was constantly on the go, with a chronic case of FOMO. I was that person who knew someone in every circle—the personification of six degrees of separation.

It was a defense mechanism.

Growing up, my sensitivity made me an easy target for bullies. To give you a sense of how easy a target I was, my first bully was a kindergartener. I was in the third grade. I was intrigued by my pint-size preliterate persecutor, who possessed a bewilderingly sophisticated insult-laden vocabulary for her age.

Common sense would have told me to shrug my shoulders and walk away. Instead, I froze, fixated, as if she knew the *real* truth about me. She was a foreshadowing of bullies to come, all of whom circled my vulnerabilities like vultures, foraging on my fragile self-esteem as if it were a delicacy.

I became so adept at anticipating threats that perception became reality. I imagined that everyone was judging me as too much—or perhaps not enough. The friendships that faded without explanation or closure impacted me more than those that remained. I became fixated on developing as many friendships as I could as a buffer for those I would inevitably lose. Acceptance was worth exhausting my energy to please others. I anticipated their needs, reframing my own as nonessential and irrelevant. I shed my preferences and hid my flaws to fit into a mold of perfection, bartering authenticity for approval.

I would only understand why several decades later.

One feature of ADHD is hypersensitivity. Criticism, insults, and rejection can feel intensely painful and difficult to regulate. This explains why I would avoid conflict and go out of my way to ensure that everyone else was happy. I would talk myself out of things I wanted with all my heart, not just because I feared failure but also because I wasn't sure if I could handle success.

Healing from this has not been a linear journey. All the things I have done to protect myself from pain felt logical to me, so they were difficult to unravel. They still *felt* safe.

It takes hard work to shift deep-seated beliefs.

I can honestly say, however, that it has been worth it. I can see more of my authentic self, and I am protective of her. I have become a more honest communicator, finding the courage to express my preferences and needs even when it's difficult and not what others want to hear.

The boundaries I have established don't shut people out—they protect my ability to connect without abandoning myself.

I now prioritize being in community with people who have mutual values rooted in respect because I know I am worthy of receiving what I so generously give. This desire to have the love that goes out in the world reciprocated is something we all desire. We deserve a community we can count on, where we uplift and affirm each other, ensuring there is always someone to fix our crown when our self-perception gets distorted.

We activate compassion in one another.

Because humans are not meant to journey alone.

## A Visualization Practice

Imagine you are standing outside on a dark evening, far away from city lights. A few people have gathered for what promises to be an incredible night under the stars.

The air is crisp as you walk onto a patio where others are beginning to take their seats. As the sky darkens, a single star appears above. You are handed a blanket and a thermos to fill with decaf coffee, cocoa, or tea. You settle into your own seat and look up toward the sky. You are greeted by a vast array of stars, far too many to count. They glitter like diamonds against the navy sky. You see several shooting stars darting across, as if chasing one another.

People start to point out different constellations. Someone quickly recognizes the Big Dipper, noting that it looks like a spoon or ladle. With some guidance, the group locates additional points forming Ursa Major, or "Big Bear." A while later, someone points out the Little Dipper, part of Ursa Minor, or "Little Bear."

Next, someone points out the three dots in a line that make up Orion's Belt. Together, you make out the stars that identify his body, shield, and sword. Several people laugh at the revelation that Orion's shoulder is a star named Betelgeuse, or "Giant's

Shoulder." "Don't call it three times, or he'll appear!" someone shouts. So, of course, someone does.

The group erupts with laughter, and your heart is filled with joy. As the laughter settles down, a collective sense of reverence falls upon the gathering, as if everyone were transfixed by the starry sky that watches over our existence.

Time seems to stand still. You think about the first star you noticed in the sky tonight. Now, it is one of countless stars that form constellations.

We were designed to be in community with others, connected to the broad expanse of humanity like constellations in the sky.

## Safety on Your Journey

As we focus on relationships with others, it is important to acknowledge that there are some relationships that may not feel emotionally safe to explore right now. If this is the case for you, please take precautions. It may be wise to begin your exploration with less complex relationships. Please consider your unique circumstances and needs when exploring the practices shared in this chapter. Consider debriefing what you observe with a trusted friend, family member, or professional.

What steps can you take to ensure your safety as you explore relationships in your life? Are there any boundaries that will be helpful to put into place?

### RETREAT RESET

Take a moment to picture the kind of people with whom you have (or would like to have) a nurturing connection. This might include

- People you look forward to spending time with, whether it's sharing a hobby, enjoying a meal, or simply relaxing and having a good time

- People who cheer you on throughout your journey, offering encouragement and support
- People who have had experiences similar to yours, who can relate to what you're going through, and who provide solidarity, helpful tips, and a sense of common humanity
- People who are a source of wisdom, offering valuable insights and perspective on your journey based on their own experiences
- People who will challenge you to grow, pushing you toward personal development and new horizons

Now, envision these people as a constellation of stars connected to you, even when you feel you are the only star in the sky. This is your support squad—a group of individuals ready to stand by your side, guiding, supporting, and inspiring you as you continue on your path.

If you have them, keep them close and nurture them. If you want more connections like this, let's build your squad.

MINI-RETREAT #1:
## CONQUER ISOLATION THROUGH CONNECTION

### The Case for Connection

We all share a common need for connection—to be part of a supportive community that makes us feel welcome and accepted. As Brené Brown states in her book *Daring Greatly*, "Connection is why we're here. We are hardwired to connect with others, it's what gives purpose and meaning to our lives, and without it there is suffering."[1]

For some, this is achieved through a few deep, meaningful relationships. Others benefit from a variety of connections, ranging from a close-knit circle built on trust to casual acquaintances with whom they share diverse interests. Healthy relationships can positively impact our daily lives and benefit our health, influencing both our health behaviors and our ability to cope with mental health challenges.

We also benefit from periods of solitude. It is important to distinguish this from social isolation, which can be harmful.

### Solitude Versus Social Isolation

Solitude is more than a preference for being alone. It can be used intentionally to retreat from the outside world to rest, gain clarity and insight, or connect with a higher power. Introspective practices may help cultivate positive emotions such as peace or joy.

Social isolation, on the other hand, is a lack of connection. One can feel socially isolated even when they're not alone. For instance, someone could have thousands of followers on social media but few meaningful connections. Loneliness and social isolation can negatively impact one's health, increasing risk of physical and mental health conditions and premature death.[2]

### Isolation Through an Intersectional Lens

In a 2022 survey of US adults, one in three reported experiencing loneliness and one in four reported not having adequate social or emotional support.[3] This was particularly pronounced among marginalized racial and ethnic groups. Factors that increase the risk of isolation and loneliness include poor mental or physical health, experiences of discrimination, inadequate access to resources, living alone, immigration status, age (both younger and older adults are at increased risk), having a low income, being a member of the LGBTQIA+ community, living in a rural population, and being a victim of domestic violence.[4]

"The Iceberg of Despair" is how a friend of mine once described the internal struggles faced by Black women. Our closest friends may not see the depth of our struggles. We celebrate each other's wins, but when we fall, we often fall hard and alone.

We admonish one another to check on our strong friends, but struggle with this when we are the ones who need to be checked on. We hesitate to let our friends in, not wanting anyone else to experience the depth of our pain.

This hesitation is exemplified in the tragic stories of women like Cheslie Kryst, a former Miss USA, lawyer, and Entertainment Tonight correspondent. She was brilliant, beautiful, confident, and accomplished, and she also struggled with mental health challenges. Having survived a suicide attempt earlier in her life, Cheslie not only had committed to improving her own mental health but also became an advocate for others. She worked with a therapist and implemented coping practices.

Cheslie fought valiantly to do the "right things," but as her struggles intensified, she did not want to burden those who loved her. She began to isolate herself from her closest friends. It was only in her final text to her mother, who was her best friend, that her loved ones would come to know how much pain she had masked. Cheslie's mother, April Simpkins, is now a mental health advocate. She fulfilled Cheslie's final wish to publish her book, *By the Time You Read This*, ensuring that her story would live on to help others.[5]

Black women learn from a young age to stay on guard. We are ever mindful that we are being watched and scrutinized differently, even at the highest levels—whether it's Oprah Winfrey shopping for a handbag in Switzerland or a Supreme Court justice going through her confirmation process. I've seen similar patterns in my research on Black staff in higher education, where participants reported poor treatment and feeling "replaceable and isolated . . . never enough."[6]

We are so used to keeping our guard up in different spaces that we struggle to reach out when we need help. Perhaps we don't want to put a strain on anyone or risk being rejected or disappointed. We dig deeper into busyness on the surface while plunging emotionally underneath. The programming we have received to "keep it together" and continually prove our worthiness is internalized to our core.

This is why I am such a staunch advocate for having a support squad. We all need people who understand and honor our experiences. It's crucial to learn how to let someone into a space that we rarely allow ourselves to occupy, to break the cycle of silent suffering.

## The Case for Connection

An insistence on figuring things out on our own can lead to enduring our pain alone when we don't have to. If we are not careful, a few days can turn into an extended period of flying under the radar. Sometimes, the challenges we face are too heavy for us to carry on our own. It is helpful to have a trusted network of friends who can relate to our struggles and will respond to the warning signs that we need support.

You deserve to have connections that have the capacity to honor your humanity and vulnerability. This might include finding a trusted friend, family member, or therapist.

If you have any feelings of resistance related to asking for help, I can relate. However, every one of us, no matter how accomplished or strong we are, needs connection and support. We all have areas in which we struggle, and having people who are strong where we are weak can help us examine our challenges from a different perspective, or connect us to the resources we need.

### REFLECTION

1. How can you tell the difference between when you are seeking solitude and when you are experiencing isolation?

2. Who are the people in your life you would consider part of your squad? How do you support each other? If this is

not something you currently have but want to build, we will focus on this as we move into the next retreat.

## MINI-RETREAT #2:
# ASSESS YOUR CURRENT LINEUP

### Key Positions in Your Support Squad

How would you define who you consider to be a friend, family, or an acquaintance? Social cohesion is an indicator of how strong your relationships are and the extent to which you experience belonging in community with others. In this section, we will reflect on your current relationships. I will suggest three tiers you can use as a guide, but feel free to adjust them as needed. It may be helpful to use your journal as you reflect on each tier.

#### Top Tier: Your Closest Connections

First, consider your top circle. These are people you're especially close to—family members or chosen family who consistently show up for you, who provide reliable support, and with whom you share the strongest trust. You feel safe being vulnerable with them. These are the relationships you treasure the most and are willing to invest significant energy to nurture. Your closest connections may or may not include family, best friends, and romantic relationships; organize them as it makes sense to you.

#### Second Tier: Stable Friendships

The second tier may be larger than the first. These are people with whom you have a strong bond but perhaps would not share all aspects of your life. You are willing to nurture these relationships, but you don't invest as much time and energy in maintaining them as you do in the first tier.

### Third Tier: Acquaintances

The final tier includes your larger social network. These people are part of the fabric of your everyday life, past or present. You may have attended school together, currently work together, have shared hobbies or interests, or live in the same community. They are valued connections but are not as deep as the prior two tiers.

## Explore Your Relationships

For the purposes of this chapter, we will focus on your top two tiers. Consider how the friendships you have identified align with your needs, values, and interests. What is the glue, or common bond, that holds your relationship together? Examples include

- shared life experiences (e.g., life stage, cultural background, common interests)
- shared contexts (e.g., workplace, church, community)
- ability to provide insight into life experiences (e.g., work, faith)
- shared goals or values
- long-standing connections (e.g., people you have known all your life)
- those you enjoy spending time with, even if you don't have a lot in common

Each person plays a unique role in your life. For example, some help nurture your resilience and provide perspective. Some are wonderful at providing advice and emotional support, helping you stay grounded. Others might remind you to live in the moment, savor positive experiences, and be grateful for what you have. Still others encourage you to evolve and take risks.

Some people may play multiple roles, but no one should be expected to address all of them. I recognize parts of myself in

## Roles

Here are a few roles you might find helpful to organize your squad:

1. **Connector:** Helps you stay connected to your community. They may invite you to gatherings or make it a point to reach out to you regularly.
2. **Motivator:** Encourages you and affirms your worth. You find yourself feeling energized after spending time with them.
3. **Problem solver:** Helpful in exploring potential solutions to your problems, developing a strategy, or navigating a complex situation.
4. **Rock:** Provides stability and unwavering support in tough times. They are a consistent presence in your life and know how to speak to you when you are struggling.
5. **Mentor:** Generously shares their life experience and insights to help nurture your growth.
6. **Expert:** Has specialized knowledge or skills in an area that is of interest to you.

each area, and I have to be careful about how I express them in any given friendship. In the past, I tried to be everything to everyone—and in the end, it only meant that I was nothing to myself.

It is important to think about the areas in which you are naturally strong and those where you need more support. Ideally, your friendships provide an opportunity for a stable exchange of each other's strengths, benefiting everyone as a result.

A strong squad is built on mutual respect and shows up for each other, ensuring no one has to go through life alone.

## REFLECTION

1. Of the positions described, which are filled by your current support squad in a way that meets your needs?
2. Where do you see gaps in your support squad?

MINI-RETREAT #3:

# CURATE YOUR ROSTER

## Preserving Flow in Your Most Important Relationships

As you complete the reflections throughout this chapter, you are developing a living document that captures your evolving needs and helps you communicate intentionally with your support squad.

Now, let's use a critical lens to explore your current approach to communication and boundaries in relationships.

### Effective Communication

Communication is the most important element in any relationship you value and wish to maintain. Honest communication facilitates understanding and helps address conflicts when they arise.

Consider your preferred communication style and how it compares to that of those close to you. Do you understand and respect their communication needs? Can you discern when they're seeking solutions or just need a listening ear? What are your expectations about time spent together? Some friendships thrive with monthly check-ins, while others prefer daily contact.

Be aware of your emotional capacity and communicate it to avoid feeling overwhelmed. These conversations aren't easy, but they are essential for building healthy relationships that honor the needs of all parties involved.

Some conflict is inevitable, and our ability to navigate it determines the future of our relationships. Through trial and error, I've learned that avoiding difficult conversations often leads to inner resentment, misunderstandings, and heightened conflict. Conversations become increasingly awkward as both parties walk on eggshells, reluctant to share their true feelings. Rather than risk hurting each other, we let our feelings build up over time and fester.

While having an honest and respectful conversation can be challenging, it's often the best way to clear the air. I find it helpful to reflect on what happened and how it affected me. I also prepare myself for the possibility that the other person may see the situation differently and might be disappointed by what I share. This latter part always made me reluctant to have these conversations—I have had to learn that what others feel is not my responsibility, nor is it under my control.

However, taking the risk to be honest while making space for the other person's perspective has given many of my relationships the opportunity to heal and evolve. We're often able to hear each other out, address the communication rift, and move forward. Sometimes, it doesn't unfold the way I would have hoped, and I have to accept when a relationship has come to an end. It's hard to let go when it's not my choice. However, I have learned how to give myself closure. I do this by accepting reality and taking time to reflect on how I feel and what steps I might need to take in order to heal.

Remember that we're always learning about each other and ourselves. We'll be working on our communication skills for as long as we live in relationships with others. It's helpful to reflect on areas where you can grow, such as building skills in assertiveness, active listening, or empathy.

## Boundaries

As we discussed in chapter 2, establishing boundaries can be challenging. We might believe we should push through discomfort to keep the peace or avoid being seen as difficult. However, boundaries are a matter of respecting and protecting ourselves.

Healthy boundaries are a crucial part of maintaining positive, supportive relationships. They allow you to be intentional about your preferences and clear about how you wish to be treated. For example, do you prefer to keep certain parts of your life private?

The hardest part of boundaries is upholding them. It's not enough to say, "This is my boundary!" if nothing changes when it is disrespected. Without consequences, others will learn that they do not have to honor them.

You have the right to establish and uphold boundaries that protect your well-being and sense of worth. When these are violated, take it seriously. Be mindful of your limits when someone repeatedly fails to take accountability or address issues. Know when it is time to walk away and make room for new, more nurturing connections.

## Identify the Hustle

Oprah Winfrey credits Maya Angelou with one of her greatest life lessons: "When people show you who they are, believe them the first time."[7] Having been disappointed on several occasions in a relationship, Ms. Angelou encouraged Oprah to conclude from people's bad actions that they could not be trusted, rather than continuing to blame them for their bad behavior and waiting for them to change.

In the context of our relationships, the hustle can often appear as a flashing red flag that we dress up as green until we can no longer ignore it.

The hustle may become more visible as you experience strain in your relationships. Over time, burnout can occur as a result of a lack of reciprocity, mutual support, effective communication, or security in the relationship. You may experience a growing sense of apathy or difficulty feeling enthusiasm or hopefulness about the future. Relationship burnout can contribute to increasingly feeling disconnected, experiencing decreased intimacy, and, in some cases, infidelity.

For relationships that are not aligned with this current stage of your life or are no longer healthy, you will consider where you need to have difficult conversations, set boundaries, or let go. Watch for signs such as these:

- You're doing all the work to maintain the relationship.
- They are disrespectful toward you or others.
- Your interactions deplete your energy or distract from your goals.
- They display toxic or unhealthy behavior.

Abuse is never justifiable. If you are experiencing abuse, take appropriate and immediate action to seek safety and support. When we rationalize or dismiss unhealthy behaviors, we may be vulnerable to greater harm.

## Know Where to Let Go

If you are moving into a new season of your life or have experienced a significant shift, you may realize that your needs have changed. It is important to honestly and effectively communicate your needs as you are able, also taking into account the needs of the other person. However, not all of your relationships will be able to adapt and evolve in the ways you need to be supported.

In this case, you may need to explore changing the nature of the relationship (i.e., moving it to a different tier) or decide to let go. If we realize that we are at the end of a relationship, it can be very difficult to be honest with the other person. We might feel bad about disappointing or rejecting them. However, it is not realistic for us to expect that others will be happy with every decision we make.

We have to allow them to have agency in their response.

It is more important to act with truth and sincerity and be willing to take accountability for our actions than to watch things fall apart haphazardly because we did not have the courage to be honest.

When we withhold our truth, we dishonor ourselves.

## Cultivate Flow

Regularly reflect on your support squad to maintain the quality of your relationships. Recall how you assessed your lineup in mini-retreat #2 in this chapter. This is a practice you will want to repeat as needed in future seasons of your life; continue to look for the gaps and assess the quality of your current connections. Are they respectful, healthy, and reciprocal? Do they contribute to your personal growth? Have you cultivated a support squad that serves your unique needs and aligns with your values?

Nurturing meaningful relationships requires effort. Even healthy relationships have challenges and need maintenance. Commit to being a good friend if you want to have good friends.

### Expanding Your Social Circle

Consider making space for new connections as a proactive way to honor your needs as you evolve. Options to explore new opportunities for connection include

- deepening existing relationships with family, friends, or acquaintances
- joining groups with similar experiences, values, or interests (e.g., cultural activities, hobbies, spiritual practices, concerts, sports events, community events, support groups)

- attending social events, mixers, or happy hours with current friends
- meeting people online (but be intentional about the type of connection you seek)

Remember that new relationships require effort to build and maintain. When it comes to creating new connections, aim to take a sustainable approach.

Quality over quantity.

### Preparing for Emergencies and Mental Health Challenges

The best time to think about the support you need during an emergency or challenging time is now—before it is needed.

If you have had previous struggles, reflect on what you might have learned about yourself from these experiences. What were some of your triggers or signs of distress? Who are the people—from friends and family to trusted professionals—you can turn to for help?

In my own life, prior seasons of depression have taught me the importance of letting my friends in. I didn't know I had the capacity to isolate as much as I did. However, I truly believed that I would be a burden or bring everyone down. I'm extremely grateful to have friends who have walked similar journeys. We now know that we take turns—we are there to support each other so that no one is a burden.

We give permission to ask each other hard questions about our mental health. We talk about what signs to look out for when one of us is struggling. Some of us go silent, while others hide behind humor. Some of us don't want to eat at all, while others turn to impulsive eating, shopping, or travel to numb or escape the pain. We talk about who to reach out to if more help is needed. It is not in our power to save one another. If one of us is struggling with seeking professional help, we are there to support them, reminding them they are not alone.

Those of us who have walked in seasons of loss, pain, and grief know that there is no right thing to say. Nothing will erase or replace the hurt. What we need is each other's presence and to not be forgotten in the rubble of what happened to us. We help each other to breathe again, to remember pieces of ourselves that we lost. We learn together how to move forward.

This isn't easy work. It is important to create positive memories and experiences to serve as a buffer in the hard times. Ongoing attention to nurturing your relationships in good times and bad can help make them stronger and more meaningful.

### REFLECTION

1. What might your ideal support squad look like in the future? With this intention in mind, what can you do today to start nurturing this vision?

2. What role do you believe you play on the support squads of your most important relationships? Consider sharing this with one of your trusted connections and asking for their feedback.

## An Inclusive Approach to Wellness

Consider exposing yourself to people with a diverse range of experiences and backgrounds. Researchers found the highest levels of perceived connectedness and life satisfaction among those who had diverse friend groups, where 50 percent of their friends differed from them in terms of age, race, education, or income. Such friendships help to cultivate understanding, respect, and empathy for people who are different from you.[8] For example, intergenerational connections help us see different perspectives, inform how we want to evolve, and remind us to stay young at heart. Take time to educate yourself and learn from others. Accept that you might say the wrong thing or make a mistake—and be willing to take accountability and move forward from it.

Start with exploring what you have in common and connect from a place of humanity. I notice in my classes that students are very reluctant to discuss religions or racial or ethnic groups that differ from their own because they don't want to offend anyone. I try to create common ground by drawing attention to cultural elements from various groups to help reinforce that many values, such as caring for our communities, are shared.

We also explore what makes each culture special and unique, such as the rituals and foods they embrace. I want them to hear from the voices of each culture what gives them joy or pride long before we discuss their challenges. My students become more comfortable as they begin to realize how much we all have in common.

As we learn to celebrate what unites us, we become more tolerant and understanding of our differences, strengthening our sense of connectedness to one another.

# Self-Preservation

*Navigating Your Roles*

Think of each part of your life, from your roles and responsibilities to your hobbies and passions, as plants in a garden. Each plant symbolizes a unique aspect of yourself, and together they create a vibrant ecosystem. To thrive, your garden needs sunlight, soil, and water, which symbolize your self-care practices, the support you receive from others, and the resources available in your environment.

Your garden's vitality depends on the flow of water and sunlight—your connection to your community and the world around you. By nurturing relationships, seeking mentors, and embracing new opportunities, you enrich your soil. Just as soil benefits from rest between seasons, so do you. These breaks allow you to prepare for new growth.

Weeds, pests, and harsh weather symbolize life's challenges. Pruning and weeding create optimal conditions for growth; similarly, you take action to address stressors that might lead to burnout. Like a fence keeps pests out, you put boundaries in place to protect yourself from toxic elements in your roles, relationships, or environments. You acknowledge when it's time to let go, seeking the help you need to heal and move forward.

Managing a thriving garden requires discernment, selecting plants that are appropriate for the season and spacing them out to avoid overcrowding. You are intentional about planning your life in line with your values and what matters most to you, such as caring for family or advancing your career. You protect space for pursuits that energize you, nurture your sense of self, bolster your resilience, and enable you to use your resources to positively impact the lives of others.

You recognize your limits, avoiding taking on more than you have the capacity to nurture. Each season, you learn how to adapt to the unexpected and conserve your energy to ensure that your garden continues to flourish.

With this image in mind, reflect on your garden:

- What fruit do you want to plant? (i.e., what is most important to you in this season?)
- What weeds can you see? (i.e., what factors might compromise your well-being?)
- What fences or fertilizers might you need to use? (i.e., what helps protect and promote your sense of well-being?)

These questions serve as a gateway to this chapter's focus on how your roles and responsibilities impact your well-being. The mini-retreats in this chapter are designed to help you gain insight into what helps you find fulfillment in your roles and what factors might contribute to harm.

## RETREAT RESET

Take a moment to anchor yourself in this present moment. Feel the connection between your body and a surface, whether it is your feet touching the ground or your back leaning against a chair.

Pause to take a gentle breath, allowing your chest to softly expand and contract. Now turn your mind to your current reality, allowing it to come into view. Notice the roles, responsibilities, and other factors that contribute to a sense of overwhelm and uncertainty in your life. Identify the parts that feel beyond your control and create strain as you try to stay afloat. Simply acknowledge how you feel as they come to mind, without judging them.

Step back from this scene as if you are now hovering above it so that you are able to see with the benefit of added perspective. Notice the forces that are piling more and more on your plate. Overwhelming expectations in your roles. Survival. The need to care for others (and yourself). The efforts you undertake to ensure your job is secure, so that you can move ahead or maintain a lead that feels increasingly precarious. Perhaps there are several things that should not be your responsibility, but no one else is willing to do them. You don't feel as if you have a choice.

Now, imagine that the same forces are all here, but they cannot touch you. You have a force field that surrounds you. You are in control of what is allowed to go in or out. This protective boundary helps you be aware of your needs and priorities. It provides a safe buffer so that you will not lose sight of yourself. Here, your energy is carefully monitored so that you are conscious of when you are pouring out faster than you are replenishing. It is a process designed to protect you so that you never empty out.

Pause to take another gentle breath. Notice the rise and fall of your chest as it surrenders to this life-sustaining process. What is it that you want to feel in this space? Peace? Fulfillment? Breathe in and out, welcoming it into your reality.

How does it feel to be here? You may stay here for a moment, noting how this feels in your body. Then, welcome movement back, gently and slowly, into your body. When you are ready to move on, take a deep breath.

## MINI-RETREAT #1:
# CULTIVATE YOUR SENSE OF SELF

### Looking Beyond Your Roles

While there may be many aspects of your roles that you consider to be a part of your identity, they do not encompass all of who you are. Yet, when we meet someone, the first question we are often asked is what we do for a living.

Who are you beyond what you do? Who are you to yourself?

It is important to define ourselves apart from what we do because a time may come when we no longer have these roles or are not needed in the same way we are today. Who are we then?

Let's start with who you are *not*. You are not your thoughts, actions, roles, achievements, accolades, or proximity to perfection.

You *are* simply present in this moment, experiencing life. You are observing everything, from your thoughts to your breath to each scene explored in this book.

The reflections you have completed throughout this journey have been designed to help you cultivate a strong sense of self—your identity, perception of your worth, beliefs, personality, and values. We have developed this by exploring self-awareness and your identity (chapter 1), affirming your inherent worth and how you define purpose (chapter 2), and fostering self-compassion (chapter 3). Throughout all the chapters, we encouraged introspection, creating boundaries, and identifying your strengths. We have explored other methods of gaining insight into yourself such as therapy.

Let's talk about another key to a sense of self: cultivating your passions. Your passions are areas in which you have great interest and experience strong emotions like excitement. They might include

- what you enjoy doing for the sake of doing it (without the need to be perfect or productive)

- what helps you be present in this moment and savor life
- what replenishes your energy
- what cultivates positive emotions
- what helps you be curious, playful, creative, and innovative

Additionally, they may address one or more of the areas of well-being we explored earlier in this section.

I am passionate about many things, including reading, music, travel, exploring new cultures, and watching documentaries. These feed several of my character strengths, such as curiosity, love of learning, and appreciation of beauty and excellence.

I thrive when I incorporate these activities into my schedule on a regular basis. Sadly, they are the first to go when I am overwhelmed by my roles and responsibilities.

For example, when I first started out as a professor, I decided I didn't have time to read for pleasure. By the end of the year, I was miserable! I didn't realize how much reading helped me replenish my energy and broaden my perspective.

I decided that moving forward, I needed to protect time each day to unwind with reading, meditation, music, or other interests. Here are a few examples:

- My garden is a refuge. I like to keep it simple and low-maintenance, with plants that grow well year-round. I find it peaceful to watch bees pollinate flowers, and I draw inspiration from the beautiful colors and fragrant scents.
- Trying out new activities engages my curiosity and stretches me beyond my comfort zone. I like that I have tried things like flyboarding and surfing, even if my mind-body coordination won't let me be great at them. Daring to do things that don't come easily strengthens

my confidence and courage to take risks in other areas of my life. It reminds me that failure is not fatal; on the contrary, it means that I am brave enough to live life to the fullest. It invites me to learn, adjust, and try again.

- I am happiest when I am singing and dancing. These practices lift my spirits by helping me unpack how I feel, express my emotions, and find release. I have specific genres, songs, or playlists I listen to depending on my mood.

- Walking outdoors allows me to enjoy nature and often helps me come up with creative approaches to problems in my professional or personal life.

- Travel is my favorite way to be present in the moment. When I am flying, I feel like time has been suspended, giving me space to be deeply introspective about my life. When I am immersed in a new culture, their customs help me see life from a new perspective. I enjoy visiting other countries, but I don't have to go far to get this feeling. Engaging with different cultures within my own community can also transport me.

- Service gives me an opportunity to uplift others by leveraging my skills. I derive great satisfaction from mentorship, helping others to grow personally and professionally and achieve their goals. I also enjoy connecting people to resources that enhance their lives.

- Quiet time spent alone helps me recharge my energy. My at-home retreat practice hones my ability to hear my voice and sense my needs. Here, I can turn down the volume of the world, even if just for a few hours. If I am short on time, a few minutes of meditation or listening to solfeggio frequencies* can help reset my day.

---

*These are nine distinct repeating musical patterns, ranging from 174 Hz to 963 Hz, that can help to alleviate stress and promote relaxation.

These pursuits address my need for connection and belonging, provide opportunities for growth, and protect me from harm by helping me manage stress.

When I do take time to do these things, I am affirming that I matter, that I am worthy of spending time on myself.

These activities help establish harmony in my life by providing a buffer from my roles and responsibilities. Boundaries are an essential practice for protecting this margin in my life.

These practices are an important part of who I am, reflecting my personality, values, and interests. All of these work together to strengthen my sense of self. This helps me be resilient and confident as I navigate an uncertain world.

Your passions should be reflective of what helps you cultivate a sense of self. What works for you may be very different from the answers I provided above.

### REFLECTION

1. What passions or pursuits help you define yourself apart from what you do?
2. What helps you be present and savor life?
3. What replenishes your energy?

## MINI-RETREAT #2:
# AVOID BURNOUT IN YOUR ROLES

### Naming the Factors That Contribute to Stress and Burnout

Society often presents an idealized picture of how we should manage our lives—effortlessly juggling multiple roles, finding contentment in each of them, and if not, fearlessly forging new paths to find our bliss. The mantra "If I can do it, anyone can" creates the illusion that this is attainable for all if we only work hard enough.

We're back to the bootstraps!

It's impossible to balance work and life if we lack autonomy in our roles, lack control over our schedules, or have overwhelming workloads. Many workplaces fall short of providing job security, adequate benefits and compensation, or opportunities for growth. Personal and professional responsibilities quickly become overwhelming without support and resources.

All of this makes it difficult to do the things that replenish us—resting, devoting time to personally meaningful pursuits, and nurturing our relationships. A strong work ethic isn't enough to compensate for a broken system.

## Burnout

Burnout is killing us. Literally.

The World Health Organization estimates that each year overwork contributes to 745,000 deaths worldwide.[1] In many workplaces, overwork is the norm, essential for advancement or simply to protect one's role. When we burn the candle at both ends, it's our health and relationships that pay the price.

It doesn't have to be this way.

In professional settings, burnout is the result of the structural demands of one's role, not the individual. As we explore this concept, consider how similar pressures might arise in the contexts of caregiving, relationships, and roles in the community.

Burnout is typically characterized in three ways: emotional exhaustion, depersonalization, and a reduced sense of personal accomplishment.[2]

- *Emotional exhaustion* may manifest as feelings of overwhelm, sadness, anxiety, or fatigue.

- *Depersonalization* may look like increased cynicism or distance in your interactions with colleagues and clients.
- A *reduced sense of personal accomplishment* may mean feeling that no matter how hard you try, your efforts will never be enough, or that you no longer find your work fulfilling.

Individuals in helping professions, such as teachers and health care workers, are particularly prone to burnout. Left unaddressed, burnout can lead to serious health issues, including cardiovascular disease, insomnia, and depression, as well as job dissatisfaction and absenteeism.[3]

Another common issue among those in client-facing roles is secondary traumatic stress. This can occur when an individual is overexposed to the trauma of those they serve. Having to frequently discuss distressing details, to the point that one absorbs it, can cause a traumatic response.

Despite a growing recognition of the importance of mental health, the stigma remains pervasive in many sectors. Those in high-profile or high-stakes roles, such as doctors, executives, or pilots, may be particularly hesitant to disclose their struggles, fearing potential repercussions. In a study of pilots, reasons for being unwilling to seek out available mental health resources included distrust of the confidentiality of the reporting system and belief that there would be severe consequences for their career.[4]

It's difficult to expect those with so much to lose to lead the charge for structural change. Workplace efforts that focus on individual responsibility and occasional morale-boosting activities fall short of addressing the deeper systemic issues in organizational cultures that impede wellness.

Findings from the *2023 Work in America Survey* by the American Psychological Association highlight several of these issues. Less than one-third of workers felt their managers prioritize caring for mental health, and four out of ten people feared negative repercussions if they were to disclose their mental health status. Only one in three felt encouraged to take breaks. Unsurprisingly, more than half were dissatisfied with workplace support for mental health and well-being, and one in three intended to seek a new role the following year.[5]

As an effort to address these issues, the US Surgeon General's *Framework for Workplace Mental Health & Well-Being* highlighted five areas and underlying needs that are critical to fostering a supportive work environment. The *2023 Work in America Survey* explored how each factor impacted the well-being of American workers:

- **Protection from harm (security, safety):** One in five employees reported a toxic work environment, correlating with poorer mental health.
- **Connection and community (social support, belonging):** One in four people reported feeling isolated or lonely in the workplace. Younger employees and those with marginalized identities (Black, Hispanic, LGBTQIA+, etc.) were more likely to report their identity negatively impacted the support they received.
- **Work-life harmony (autonomy, flexibility):** One in five people were dissatisfied with the amount of control they had over how their work was structured. Three in five did not feel that their management respected boundaries around time off.
- **Mattering at work (dignity, meaning):** Most respondents felt valued and believed their work was meaningful. However, those experiencing micromanagement or a lack of meaningful work were more likely to report feeling stressed.
- **Opportunity for growth (learning, accomplishment):** Nine in ten people desired a workplace environment

that facilitated growth and accomplishment. Those who lacked opportunities for growth were more likely to report job dissatisfaction and feeling stressed.

These experiences varied widely based on factors like work environment, income, role level, marginalized identity, and workplace culture (e.g., diversity in leadership; presence of policies addressing equity, diversity, and inclusion).

## Caregiving Burnout

Burnout can also occur in the context of caregiving, which includes caring for the needs of someone else—such as children, other family members, and pets—and serving as their advocate. This is especially the case for those managing it alone or as part of the sandwich generation—balancing care for children and aging relatives while working full- or part-time. Nearly two-thirds of caregivers experience burnout, compromising their well-being. Many lack adequate support, underscoring the importance of having a village to share the load or access to online resources, such as caregiver networks and support groups.

Burnout in any area can affect all aspects of life, including relationships and health. It's possible to experience burnout in multiple areas simultaneously, extending beyond what we have explored here.

Recovery from burnout requires deep care for those affected and fostering supportive environments through systemic change. When change isn't sufficient, it may be necessary to step back from certain roles or responsibilities to recover and preserve your well-being.

Take a moment to pause. Perhaps some of what you have read here has resonated with you, or you recognize some of the signs of burnout in people in your life. The information we have discussed here is intended to foster self-awareness so that we are better equipped to detect burnout and take action. Now, we are prepared to explore strategies to promote well-being in the next retreat.

### REFLECTION

1. What support or resources do you have access to in navigating your roles and responsibilities? What support or resources do you need?
2. How do aspects of your identity and lived experiences inform how you navigate your roles?
3. Do you feel that you have experienced burnout in one or more of your roles? What was your experience like?

MINI-RETREAT #3:
## FOSTER WELL-BEING IN YOUR ROLES

### Requirements for Well-Being

We will now use the five priority areas in the US Surgeon General's *Framework for Workplace Mental Health & Well-Being* to explore how roles and responsibilities in all areas of life—such as work, family, and community—influence our well-being.[6] I've broadened two areas of the framework—work-life harmony and mattering at work—to include other roles.

- protection from harm
- connection and community
- harmony between roles, responsibilities, and personal life
- mattering
- opportunity for growth

At the center of the original framework was worker voice and equity, which we will reframe as voice and equity across all contexts of your life—the extent to which you feel you are heard and treated fairly.

Life is complex, and your experiences and preferences in each of these areas may vary from one context to the next. You may feel a strong sense of connection in your community but have concerns about overall safety. You may feel like you matter at work but have few opportunities for growth.

Some embrace the opportunity for connection at work, while others prefer to keep a low profile and maintain firm boundaries between their professional and personal lives. Two individuals may be exposed to the same environment, but the extent to which they experience harm may depend on how vulnerable they are based on their position and access to resources.

As you explore examples for each area, think about how they apply to your various roles, whether as a family member, caregiver, professional, or community member, or in your personal life as you manage various responsibilities.

## Protection from Harm

This area addresses needs for safety and security. This includes actions taken to prevent injuries and adverse health outcomes (such as burnout or illness) and to promote physical and mental well-being. In a workplace that has psychological safety, you can ask for help, take risks to create and innovate, and admit errors without fear of reprisal. Safety also means having job security; adequate compensation; support and affirmation for your identity; and protection from discrimination, harassment, or bullying.

If we do not have psychological safety in our workplace, it will affect how we show up. We will not be authentic, and we may shut down and focus on survival. If others are creating a hostile environment, and there is no accountability, it takes an emotional toll. We spend effort we could contribute to the world around us on processing situations and protecting our energy instead.

Environments with low psychological safety breed incivility. Alternatively, in a safe setting, promoting mindful self-compassion has the power to create a ripple effect. When we are kinder toward ourselves, it can affect how we treat others.

Even if we have a supportive environment, there are other factors that might make a role untenable. For example, we discussed earlier how an overwhelming workload can contribute to burnout. Another factor is inadequate resources or compensation. We also may experience harm in one part of our lives that makes it impossible to show up fully in our other roles.

During a season when I faced significant health challenges, I had to take multiple periods of disability leave. Each time I tried to resume work, I put my health at greater risk. Ultimately, I had to let go of the role and start over again. This was not easy, but it humbled me and taught me an important lesson.

No job is worth my life.

In what ways might your roles or responsibilities protect you from harm?

In what ways might your roles or responsibilities subject you to harm?

## Connection and Community

This area addresses needs for social support and belonging. It includes having supportive relationships built on trust and respect and environments that value authenticity, transparency, and collaboration.

Relationships are vital to my well-being, so I intentionally nurture them across my family, work, and community roles. But throughout my academic and professional career, I have almost always been one of few people who look like me in each context.

I call this club the "onlies or the lonelies."

When starting a new opportunity, I seek out people with shared values or experiences to build community with. And I value my connections with family and friends, as they provide encouragement and nurture a sense of belonging when I navigate environments that don't always offer these elements.

On my campus, I enjoy partnering with faculty who have similar interests across disciplines. I also like involving students so that their perspectives are considered and they have an opportunity to develop their skills and explore their interests. We also have a small but supportive community of Black faculty, staff, and students who celebrate each other.

I have found connection to be an asset when dealing with executive function challenges. Whether I am writing or doing chores, the presence of others helps me overcome the hurdles of low motivation and focus to initiate and complete tasks. Even if we are working on different things, they help me to be accountable. This is a practice known as *body doubling*. When in-person connection isn't possible, I might work with others virtually or schedule periodic check-ins to ensure I stay on task.

Without these supports, I tend to hyperfocus on one area while neglecting others or drift toward distractions that provide instant gratification. This is just one of many important accommodations in my home and work life that honor my authentic needs.

In what ways might you experience connection and feeling wanted and accepted in your roles or responsibilities?

How might you experience isolation in your roles or responsibilities or feel as if you are not wanted or accepted?

## Harmony Between Roles, Responsibilities, and Personal Life

This area addresses the need for autonomy and flexibility. This includes having independence, control over how tasks are completed, a predictable yet flexible schedule, boundaries that are respected and protected, and access to paid leave.

Even in roles with flexible schedules, work-life conflict can arise from the combination of unrealistic workloads or overwhelming responsibilities and inadequate support in other areas of life. When the workday is endless or leads into a mountain of responsibilities at home, it is challenging to prioritize one's well-being. This can impact workplace performance in turn. Structural support is needed for individuals to achieve harmony across the different roles in their lives.

What helps you experience harmony between your roles, responsibilities, and personal life?

What contributes to conflict between your roles, responsibilities, and personal life?

## Mattering

This area addresses needs for dignity and meaning. This can include receiving fair compensation and access to benefits (e.g., health care, retirement, childcare), feeling valued, understanding the significance of your role to the overall mission, having input in the organizational direction, and seeing meaningful action result from assessments of engagement, well-being, and satisfaction.

When workplace compensation does not close wage gaps or reflect the increasing costs of living, the well-being of employees and their households is compromised. No number of platitudes or amount of recognition makes up for not being able to provide for one's needs.

Parents and caregivers spend many hours doing unpaid labor, which is often undervalued and rendered invisible by our society. We turn a blind eye to the fact that most households would not function without unpaid labor. Consider if you were to outsource all of the following services: child care, pet care, meal preparation, house cleaning, transportation, grocery shopping, laundry, interior decoration, management of finances, homework assistance, mentoring and emotional support, activity and appointment planning, home maintenance and repairs, in-home health care, and chaperoning or accompanying family members to and from activities and appointments. The cost would be overwhelming and unsustainable.

In addition to the dignity of being able to care for one's needs and those of their household, it is important to experience meaning in our roles. I find deep meaning in my roles as a professor, speaker, and coach, and in my relationships with my loved ones. I try to practice character strengths such as love, honesty, integrity, teamwork, and justice in each of my roles.

This past year, I found profound meaning in caring for my grandmother in her final months of life. I was able to use my professional background to help my family navigate end-of-life care. I frequently visited her in hospice, where I instinctually began to comb her hair and do other things to affirm her worth and dignity. Although her physical presence was fading, I was not jarred because I also witnessed the spiritual transformation that was taking place. During my last visit, my mother noticed her studying a flower with all her senses, taking in its color, texture, and scent.

For years, I had worried about losing our family matriarch. However, I had lost so many family members suddenly in that time period that I appreciated for once having an opportunity to say goodbye. My recent life challenges also prepared me, pushing me beyond the limits of my own strength to lean on the faith that my grandmother and I had shared since I was a child. By the time she departed this world, her spirit was anchored inside of me.

In what ways do you feel valued in your roles and responsibilities?

How do you *not* feel valued in your roles and responsibilities?

## Opportunity for Growth

This area addresses needs for learning and accomplishment. Key elements include access to mentorships, opportunities for skill development, and clear paths for advancement; feeling a sense of accomplishment; and receiving constructive feedback in a timely manner to identify strengths and areas for growth.

I have built a strong network of mentors in my personal and professional life. I benefited from programs during college and early in my professional career that trained me to reach out for informational interviews with individuals who had experience in areas I was interested in. At my current institution, structured mentorship and clear guidelines, combined with feedback that helped me identify areas for growth, aided me in navigating the tenure track successfully. While earning tenure was a significant milestone, it took a while to sink in. Like many high achievers, I sometimes struggle to pause and savor my accomplishments. I just keep going, in search of something to improve or perfect.

I am learning to prioritize my own needs alongside serving others. I know there is no need to run the race as hard and fast as I have up until this point in my career. I now aim to set a more sustainable pace, set healthy boundaries, and identify strategies that allow me to work effectively while protecting my well-being.

Growth takes on different forms as we move through life stages. For my clients approaching retirement, we focus on legacy, impact, and preparing their successors, as well as whether they will continue professional work or focus on family and community.

What opportunities might you pursue to acquire knowledge, develop skills, advance to a new level, or feel a sense of accomplishment in your roles and responsibilities?

What obstacles stand in the way of pursuing such opportunities?

## Voice and Equity

The themes of voice and equity are the central focus of the framework. You may consider how they are relevant to your well-being in each area. For example, in the context of workplace dynamics, consider whether the perspectives and experiences of all workers are taken into account, and if there is equity in treatment and compensation.

For people of color and other marginalized groups, authenticity comes with inherent risks. We navigate prescribed roles and expectations while maintaining vigilance about our safety and security in ways that others may not ever consider. This affects how we present ourselves and navigate spaces, and it takes a toll on our physical and mental health.

Where do you feel that you are treated fairly and that your voice is heard? In what ways do you feel that you are silenced or treated unfairly?

Throughout this chapter, you have reflected on how to nurture your sense of self outside of your roles and responsibilities. You have also reflected on factors that have contributed to burnout, as well as those that have helped to promote your well-being. Now, let's take some time to think about where the hustle is showing up across your roles, where you might need to let go, and how you can create more flow.

## Identify the Hustle

Having explored your experiences in this chapter, consider the following questions in the context of your roles and responsibilities.

What factors have contributed to the hustle in your roles? Are there specific influences—from the nature of your role to your cultural upbringing or your own inner dialogue—that trigger you to go into hustle mode? When and how have your experiences of the hustle contributed to burnout?

## Cultivate Flow

What practices help you experience flow in your roles and responsibilities? This might include taking breaks, enforcing boundaries to protect your time off, taking mental health days when needed, coordinating care with other family members, or seeking respite care services.

How might cultivating your sense of self help you experience more flow? For example, what activities or interests might allow you to explore and engage in your passions outside of your roles?

What might be helpful strategies to prevent or address burnout? Consider the following:

1. What would be a warning sign for when you are heading toward burnout?
2. What would be an effective guardrail to protect your well-being? With whom do you feel safe asking for support or guidance or discussing your experiences?
3. What strategies can help you combat overwhelm in your role? How might you break projects into smaller tasks or protect time on your schedule?
4. How might you explore options in community to advocate for support to decrease the intensity of your role?

## Know Where to Let Go

In considering what you would like to let go of, focus both on factors that are under your control and on those that need to be addressed as a collective—such as standards for safety, compensation, discriminatory practices, or how roles in your organization are structured.

Which factors are under your control? In some cases, the only thing you control is how you respond. Are there unhealthy beliefs or assumptions that you need to address or release? Are there aspects of your roles or responsibilities that you need to let go of for now?

Which factors are not under your control? Examples might include your workload or schedule, and efforts such as addressing workplace policy may require collective action.

## REFLECTION

Consider what must be done at a systemic level to improve your experiences in each area:

- protection from harm
- connection and community
- harmony between roles, responsibilities, and personal life
- mattering
- opportunity for growth

## An Inclusive Approach to Wellness

There is no balance without equity.

Our access to educational and economic opportunities varies widely. Not everyone grows up in a supportive environment with resources that provide them with the safety to dream and pursue those dreams. Yet mainstream narratives often celebrate isolated success stories, perpetuating the "If I can do it, anyone can" mantra despite the systemic barriers many face.

Many people wrestle with workplace environments that pose physical or emotional harm. In cultures with low psychological safety, individuals don't feel safe taking risks, asking questions, or making mistakes, leading to disconnection due to low trust and a lack of transparency. These environments are less innovative and struggle to address problems effectively. Similarly, efforts to promote diversity and inclusion in these environments are vulnerable to budget cuts and legislative changes.

For some, there is no end to the workday. Their job descriptions and working hours are not meaningfully enforced, and as positions are eliminated, their roles expand without additional compensation. A lack of opportunities for growth stagnates ambition as workers struggle to meet their roles' demands without adequate support.

Roles that expose individuals to distress or trauma, such as those in human services, present another set of challenges. In addition to structural inefficiencies causing burnout, workers face secondary traumatic stress due to their exposure to others' trauma, highlighting a profound need for targeted support systems.

And what about those with inadequate employment or a lack of opportunities altogether? In a world where survival hinges on employment, applying to jobs that hundreds or even thousands of people are also applying to can feel more like a lottery than a meritocracy.

**Without systemic change, we are living in a world where burnout becomes an inevitability.**

Labor doesn't begin and end at the workplace. At home, strain continues when professional and personal roles blur. Caregivers juggle their families' needs, often with insufficient support, and many wrestle with toxic environments or unhealthy relationships behind closed doors.

Without systemic change, we are living in a world where burnout becomes an inevitability.

Addressing these inequities requires collective thinking and action, looking beyond individual responsibility. We must build systems that recognize and support diverse needs, fostering true inclusivity and equity.

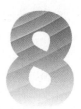

# Create Your Blueprint

*A Sustainable Plan for Your Future*

Imagine stepping into a space designed just for you, where you can rest and focus on creating your own wellness blueprint. This setting encourages exploration of what best supports your well-being, allowing you to distance yourself from daily pressures of the hustle and reconnect with yourself.

Here, it is as if time is suspended, inviting you to take things at your own pace. One afternoon spent napping and relaxing here can rejuvenate you as much as days elsewhere. You're energized by the opportunity to rest, enjoy nourishing meals, and engage in activities that bring you joy, all without financial concerns.

In this environment, you control how you interact with others and technology. You have the choice to disconnect from your phone and take a break from the constant stream of social media, news, calls, and messages, allowing you the freedom to explore solitude or connect with others as you see fit.

The space includes elements that enhance your relaxation. Choose from a variety of scents—flowers, candles, diffusers—or none at all. Your room is painted in calming colors and decorated with artwork that appeals to you. The textures of the bedding, blankets, and furniture are chosen to help you unwind. Your favorite music plays in the background, whether you prefer calming tunes or energizing beats.

What elements of this imagined space might you want to incorporate into your life? In this chapter, you will explore how to realistically address your well-being using the resources you have and create a wellness blueprint to help guide you in the future.

## RETREAT RESET

Take a few moments to settle into your body. Let the sounds around you become part of the background—there's no need to filter them out. Just breathe deeply and notice the gentle rise and fall of your chest as you turn your attention inward.

Imagine having all the resources you need at your disposal—whether it's a flexible schedule, the energy to do what you love, the ability to meet your financial needs, or a peaceful environment that helps you unwind. Notice the thoughts and feelings that surface. How does it feel to visualize a space where you're truly cared for?

What would help evoke these feelings in your daily life? Where can you address the hustle, let go of what you can, and cultivate a sense of flow? Even on the most challenging days, what small step can you take toward connection—with yourself, others, or the world around you?

Imagine taking action in the following ways, right where you are:

Affirm your worth and recognize one thing you're grateful for.

Acknowledge your thoughts and feelings, understanding they don't define you.

Pay attention to your breath and the beating of your heart, ensuring your body's needs—such as nourishment, movement, or rest—are met.

Think of one person in your support squad you can reach out to. Reflect on your passions and what fosters a sense of well-being in one of your roles.

What if these small movements created ripple effects in your daily life? What could be possible? Stay here for as long as you need. When you're ready, take a few breaths and return to your present surroundings. Now, let's continue our journey.

## MINI-RETREAT #1:
# REVIEW YOUR WELLNESS JOURNEY

### Looking Back Before Moving Forward

We are almost ready to create your personal blueprint for wellness, but first, let's review each of the areas of wellness you have already addressed on your journey.

**Chapter 1, "Cultivating Self-Awareness":** You were not designed for a life of overwhelm. You can define for yourself what wellness means to you, based on your reality, identity characteristics, and lived experiences.

**Chapter 2, "Accepting Your Intrinsic Worth":** You possess inherent worth that cannot be diminished by others or by your actions. Spiritual practices help you restore your sense of worth and connection beyond yourself. Topics we covered include faith, perspective, meaning, awe, and gratitude.

**Chapter 3, "Exploring Your Thoughts":** Your brain is unique, influencing how you think, learn, and process information. Executive dysfunction can impact skills such as decision-making, planning, organization, impulse control, emotional regulation, and task initiation and completion. We discussed beneficial practices such as noticing thought patterns and addressing cognitive distortions and limiting beliefs.

**Chapter 4, "Managing Your Emotions":** Experiencing a range of emotions—positive, negative, neutral, or mixed—is natural. We discussed the importance of self-compassion and emotional intelligence skills, which help us identify, understand, and manage our emotions, as well as respond effectively to the emotions of others. We also explored how to shift from a fixed mindset to a growth mindset.

**Chapter 5, "Flaws and All":** Your relationship with your body can be complex. As the vessel that allows you to experience life, your body is worthy simply because it exists. We discussed practices that support nourishing yourself based on your needs, preserving functionality through movement, and prioritizing rest and recovery. We also explored navigating the health care system, recovering from injury or illness, and navigating complex health issues.

**Chapter 6, "Support Squad":** Connection is vital to our well-being. A strong support squad can help us combat isolation, expose us to diverse perspectives, and offer us encouragement, instrumental support, and wisdom. We explored practices for nurturing a strong squad, such as healthy communication, setting boundaries, knowing when to let go, and building new relationships.

**Chapter 7, "Self-Preservation":** Making room for your passions helps nurture your sense of self outside of what you do for others. We explored how factors in your roles and responsibilities within your family, workplace, and community can contribute to stress and burnout. Finally, we explored practices to foster well-being, adapted from the *Framework for Workplace Mental Health & Well-Being*. These areas included protection from harm; connection and community; harmony between roles, responsibilities, and personal life; mattering; and opportunity for growth—with voice and equity centered in each area.

## REFLECTION

1. Which area is the greatest priority for you at this time?
2. How might practices in this area have a positive impact on your life?

MINI-RETREAT #2:
## HONOR YOUR REALITY

### Exploring Our Resources

We will begin this journey by exploring our current approach to using resources such as time, energy, money, environment, technology, and social support. We vary *widely* in terms of our access to resources as well as how we utilize them in our lives. So let me be clear: What we have available to us and what we are able to do is *not* a reflection of who we are or our worth.

However, we all can benefit from leveraging the resources we have with intention, ensuring our approaches and strategies align with our values and goals. We can be conscious about eradicating shame and setting boundaries that protect what we value most. Finally, we can call out and address inequities that create barriers to wellness.

### Time and Energy

According to Chandra Prescod-Weinstein, a theoretical physicist, Black feminist, and the author of *The Disordered Cosmos*, our lay concept of time has a central motive of "keeping society organized and efficient . . . [and] increasing economic productivity."[1]

Consider all of the different milestones we are pressured to accomplish by a specific age, from becoming financially independent to getting married, having children, and owning a home.

This rigid societal expectation does not take into consideration our unique needs, preferences, abilities, and varying levels of access to resources. It also disregards larger systemic factors such as the job and housing markets. So why should these milestones be considered universal?

For many, especially those managing chronic illnesses or balancing multiple roles like work and caregiving, time is a scarce resource. In the words of Kenyan poet and activist Shailja Patel, "'We all have the same 24 hours.' Use public transport? Your 24 hours are not the same as those of private jet owners. Do your own cooking, cleaning, child-raising? Your 24 hours are not the same as those of someone with a full-time domestic staff. Stop this nonsense."[2]

Time management strategies are only realistic if they work for *your* life. Adapt them as needed and give yourself permission to let go of what does not work for you.

Rather than using time as your main metric, consider how you can prioritize using your energy and other resources to live in alignment with your core values. Focus on being present in the process, not just for the outcome. Prioritize quality of life and relationships over quantity of possessions or achievements.

Self-compassion is at the core of this approach.

Some of us have unpredictable energy cycles. We *must* be compassionate with ourselves, honoring our unique needs, whether we thrive with a predictable routine or need cushion, flexibility, and spontaneity.

I used to ride the wave of adrenaline or even coerce myself using shame to get things done, but these are not helpful long-term strategies.

Now, I try to be aware of my patterns, find strategies that help, and if all else fails, be accountable when I make mistakes. When I struggle, I'm learning to be more forthcoming about the accommodations I need, such as specific guidance, a more flexible approach, frequent checkpoints, additional time, or the elimination of distractions. I often get clarity sooner and progress to my goal with greater ease and efficiency when I am willing to ask for help.

## Deeper Dive: Time and Energy Reflection

Reflect on your energy patterns and how you approach planning. Here are a few strategies that have worked for me.

1. **Assess your capacity:** It doesn't matter how much time I give a task if I don't have the energy or focus. When I create a to-do list that is out of touch with my reality, I end up putting undue pressure on myself to follow through and blame myself when I fall short. Taking time to check in with myself and reflect on my recent patterns helps me to be honest about what I can accomplish without strain.

   - You can learn about your energy patterns by noting how your energy levels fluctuate throughout the day. Reflect on how you might address your priorities during times when your energy is highest and how you might engage in rest or activities that replenish you when your energy levels are lowest. Consider that there may be days when 100 percent of your effort is consumed by survival. On those days, surviving *is* your personal best. Develop an awareness of your capacity and the boundaries needed to protect it. The time you spend in rest and leisure is vital to sustaining your ability to show up in all areas of your life.

2. **Align your actions with your values:** I am more likely to do a task when I understand how it impacts my life and the consequences if I don't do it. For example, I nourish myself in order to have energy to carry out my daily tasks. When I skip meals or forget to hydrate, I don't think as clearly and it affects every area of my life.

3. **Create a balance of structure and flexibility that works for you:** I benefit from having a schedule that helps me to do the following:

- Have a reason to wake up in the morning and something to look forward to
- Make progress toward meaningful goals by working on small, actionable tasks that provide me with a sense of accomplishment and build momentum
- Engage in activities that energize me and promote my well-being by allowing me to be active, rest, experience joy or beauty, engage in connection, or nurture hope
- Use boundaries to protect time for my priorities and ensure I have downtime for recovery

## Money

Everywhere we go, we are bombarded with advertisements and the pressure to consume. When we are struggling financially, it can seem like everyone who is posting their new cars and vacations on social media is doing well. However, appearances can be misleading. People across all income levels are dealing with financial challenges, such as student debt, business loans, costly house repairs, unexpected tax bills, or periods of unemployment or underemployment. These financial challenges can be overwhelming and negatively impact our well-being.

It's time to normalize having these conversations.

Many of us did not grow up discussing financial literacy. Even if we did, the financial landscape is constantly evolving, and we need reliable information and resources to keep up.

I became intentional about my finances after my identity was stolen at twenty-one, which tanked my credit score just as I was seeking to relocate for a job after graduate school. I had to convince someone to lease to me based on my starting salary rather than my credit score. It took years of dealing with collections to clear my name. I took control by freezing my accounts and reading library books to develop my financial literacy. I learned about creating an emergency fund and automating savings for future goals.

However, years later, I still struggled to justify spending, even on necessities like groceries. I turned to budgeting apps to learn how to plan my spending in alignment with my priorities. By budgeting even small amounts for giving, what I call "pocket philanthropy," I found a way to make a meaningful impact in my community without waiting to be in an ideal financial state.

### Deeper Dive: Financial Reflection

Reflect on your patterns regarding money. Think about your current financial mindset and what informs your approach to money.

Here are four important strategies to consider moving forward:

1. **Develop financial literacy:** Identify topics to learn about that will help you improve your skills with managing money. Some examples include setting up a budget, investing, saving for short- and long-term goals, and dealing with debt. This knowledge will empower you to navigate financial challenges confidently.

2. **Set up a budget:** There are a wide range of tools, from apps to spreadsheets, to help you monitor your spending. Try several out to see what works best for you. Create categories that are aligned with your values and reality. Come up with an ongoing plan to review transactions to understand your spending patterns and make adjustments to your budget as needed. This will help you have more clarity and control over your financial situation.

3. **Monitor and protect your credit:** Regularly check your credit report to spot potential fraud or errors. Familiarize yourself with the fraud alert process for your accounts. If you use credit cards, find one that will not hold you financially responsible for fraud that is under review. Be sure to check your bank and card statements on a regular basis for fraudulent activity, as sometimes there is a limited time frame in which you can report such transactions.

4. **Create financial boundaries to protect yourself:** It can be difficult to say no to others, whether you're declining a social invitation that's outside your budget or turning down a request for a loan. Others may not fully understand or respect your financial situation and priorities. You have several options for how you can deal with this, from saving up over time for a fund that's dedicated to special activities to deciding on a set amount of money you're willing to spend in these areas each month. Whatever you choose, ensure it does not compromise your own financial needs in the short- or long-term. Reflect on past experiences and future goals to guide your decisions.

In my personal practice, I am proactive about incorporating wellness into my monthly budget by funding categories such as medical care, routine self-care activities (e.g. fitness, massages) alongside long-term goals like vacations. Your financial journey is unique, and your worth is not defined by monetary success. Be intentional in using the resources you have access to to promote your well-being and positively impact the lives of others.

## Environment

Whether at home, work, or out in the community, the environments you navigate on a daily basis impact the extent to which you experience safety and comfort, feel energized, engage in connection, and are able to focus, be productive, or rest. Your approach to how you navigate your environment is informed by your needs, your interests, and the resources available to you.

Consider how you can take an intentional approach to curating and navigating the spaces in which you live, work, and socialize.

### Home

In the best of circumstances, our home environment is our safe space from the world. If the amount of privacy or space you have isn't ideal, consider what *is* under your control that might help you support your well-being.

I have learned to put my daily wellness routine on autopilot by ensuring my home is stocked with the items I need. For groceries, we maintain a list of fruits, vegetables, protein sources, and snacks that we enjoy on an ongoing basis. This makes it easy to do a focused grocery run or order them online for pickup. Either approach is better than the hours I used to spend comparing prices per ounce.

One of the hardest things for me regarding my home environment has been accepting help in areas where I need support. For years, I resisted hiring someone to help because I believed I should be able to do everything on my own. However, I understand that this is a matter of finding someone who is skilled in an area that I am not and fairly compensating them for their help.

Some angels have wings, and others are professional organizers and cleaners.

When I was first diagnosed with kidney disease, an organizer helped me make sense of my clutter, find the items I loved, and let go of others that had fulfilled their purpose or were no longer meeting my needs. Together, fueled by snacks and good music, we worked at my pace, creating order by finding systems that worked for the new rhythms my life needed.

My favorite part about the process was that there was no shame. A good professional is very skilled in what they do and is not there to judge you. They want to help you feel more comfortable and at ease in your living space.

I have had similar experiences over the years with cleaners who made quick work of the tasks I find difficult and lifted my spirits as they restored my living space. From these experiences, I've learned not to morally judge myself based on my ability to carry out household tasks.

Hiring services requires saving and planning, but for me it is a crucial part of maintaining a living space that supports my health and productivity. If this is outside your budget, consider asking a close friend over to help you organize your space. None of us can do it all by ourselves.

### Workplace

In many workplaces, wellness is considered in the context of strategies like having an ergonomic setup personalized to your needs. Sure, this is an important part of ensuring your safety and comfort, which in turn influences productivity, but there is so much more to consider, especially for those who need specific accommodations.

To support my executive functioning skills, I find it helpful to incorporate movement into my day, and I have a few items on my desk that allow me to engage my senses or find novelty. My health care team also constantly reminds me to be mindful of my posture and take breaks to stretch.

If I need a change of scenery while working from home, I will switch furniture or rooms. Occasionally, I will work from a co-working space or a café. On campus, I move between my office, classrooms, the library, outdoor spaces, and other communal areas. This makes it likely that I will interact with different groups of people, a part of my work that I enjoy.

If I am working alone, I use headphones to listen to music or sit where there is some background noise—the right level of stimulation helps me stay focused. When teaching, I aim to make classes engaging by doing interactive activities and exposing students to different centers and resources on campus.

### Public Spaces

When I am in other settings, I am mindful that I can't always control my environment. Fortunately, I have found some helpful ways to manage my sensory needs and avoid overstimulation. In crowded settings, I use earplugs that allow me to hear nearby conversations while tuning out loud noises. I also carry headphones for when I am alone. If I am at a conference, I try to leave every few hours and go outside to meditate, have a meal, and allow my body to reset. When I travel, I do extensive research to ensure I have comfortable transportation and quiet accommodations. When shopping, I gravitate toward stores that are well-lit and spacious and try to go when they are less crowded.

Nature can also provide an escape, inviting us to leave our stress behind and be present as we fully engage our senses in its beauty. Whether I am hiking, walking on the beach, or admiring a waterfall, I savor these moments. I capture mental images that I can recall later to experience joy and revive my hope during challenging times. When I am not able to visit my favorite settings, I try to incorporate nature into my daily routine by going for a walk or stepping outside to look at the sun in the sky, which always helps me regain perspective. I also try to interact with nature in my home environment. I can look outside my windows and see hummingbirds (typically fighting over the feeder) or bees pollinating our African blue basil plants. On quiet days, I can hear parrots flying overhead—according to local legend, they escaped from a pet store and now roam our neighborhoods freely.

Third spaces—settings outside of your home and work where you can interact with others, such as parks, libraries, and cafés—provide additional opportunities for relaxation and community engagement. This is especially helpful for those who do not have control over how their environment is organized, lack sufficient space, or need more social interaction. A change of scenery can help reduce stress and provide inspiration.

### Deeper Dive: Environment Reflection

Assess the environments you interact with to understand whether they support your needs. Identify small changes you can make on your own or where you might need to advocate for support, such as with sensory challenges in workplaces and other environments you don't have complete control over. Identify third spaces that can support your well-being.

The following strategies have been helpful for me:

1. **Clarify the purpose of your space:** Determine the primary intention of each environment. Is it meant to be a calming area for relaxation, a productive workspace, or a place to inspire creativity? This can help you tailor everything from furniture to lighting, artwork, and colors to meet your needs.

2. **Personal function:** You can decorate your environment with elements that are functional in meeting your needs while reflecting your personality and interests. Seek out textures and colors that you enjoy and include items that allow you to foster an emotional connection with your space. For example, the items I use to decorate my dining table and the artwork I have in my home evoke positive emotions when I see them. I have collected simple art pieces from local artists throughout the African diaspora, from Ghana to Brazil, Cuba, and Nicaragua. Each piece reminds me of a specific stage of my life and reinforces pride in my heritage.

3. **Third spaces:** Explore public places that fulfill needs such as focus, connection, or the novelty of new experiences. Consider your sensory needs as you navigate environments that are not under your control, from lighting to noise, smell, or crowds.

4. **Organize your way:** Honor the way in which you need to organize or clean. Explore what helps you get through tasks, such as playing music, listening to podcasts, or talking to someone while you clean. You also can consider focusing on the task as a mindfulness practice. Don't hesitate to seek assistance if you need it. Free resources include online guides and videos that provide tips and guidance. Ask a friend over to help or to simply serve as a body double. Look for practical solutions that fit your lifestyle.

Remember, a supportive environment is not about achieving perfection but about curating or finding spaces that support your needs. Approach this process with curiosity and flexibility, understanding that what is ideal for you may change over time. The aim is to feel safe and supported in your environment so that you can recharge and focus on what matters most.

## Technology and Other Resources

In today's digital age, technology and social media are integral to our daily lives. They offer numerous opportunities for connection, learning, and self-improvement but can have both positive and adverse effects on well-being.

On one hand, technology can be a powerful tool for learning information and managing your wellness practice. For example, AI has been a game changer in helping me create systems to support my life, such as turning my notes from various health appointments into a comprehensive monthly update for my health care team. It is also a wonderful sounding board when I am fleshing out new ideas. An ethical approach to the use of AI balances its benefits with its limitations and risks, ensuring it is used in a responsible manner and its results are reviewed for accuracy.

But excessive use of technology can compromise our well-being. Hours spent craning our necks downward, hunching our shoulders forward, and scrolling with our thumbs takes a toll. Although we know the importance of taking breaks, our minds are fully immersed in a greater battle.

Many of the devices and platforms we use were created to hook us, providing us with boosts of dopamine that make us feel good. This becomes self-reinforcing, leading us to continually seek immediate gratification through doomscrolling.

In her article "The Elite College Students Who Can't Read Books," Rose Horowitch discusses how smartphones have made it increasingly difficult to engage with less stimulating tasks. As psychologist Daniel Willingham notes in the article, the distraction provided by smartphones has "changed expectations about what's worthy of attention. . . . Being bored has become unnatural."[3]

Technology is a major asset in the work that I do, so I want to be careful to encourage you to find a balance that works for you. We can set routines and craft environments that wire us to address the stress on our bodies before damage is done. This might look like setting alarms to work in blocks that alternate with breaks for stretching, walking, and hydration. It is helpful to learn signs of strain in your body and devise strategies to address them. If I work for longer than one hour at my computer or phone, I might feel okay in the moment, but my arms and eyes will suffer later in the day. The longer I work, the more I need breaks to rest my eyes and restore flow to my arms and other parts of my body.

Social media can be a wonderful tool for connection and community building. However, it can be wielded in ways that promote surface-level connection or drive division. In my own life, I try to find a balance with social media. I love using it to inspire others, interact with people all around the world, and learn new ideas. I also find it helpful to take periods away from social media, whether to hear my own voice more clearly, incubate new ideas, or recover from overstimulation. I try to reflect on the impact that exposure to disturbing content has on my well-being.

We are subject to algorithms that are increasingly effective in fostering tribalism—dividing rather than uniting us. It is important to be mindful of how we can use social media as a tool while protecting ourselves from agendas that don't have our best interests at heart. Helpful boundaries might include

- taking breaks from specific platforms
- blocking people who are disrespectful
- filtering out content that is disturbing or irrelevant
- being mindful of how much time you spend on platforms

Meaningful connections, whether in person or online, help foster positive emotions and are part what makes life fulfilling. Remember to value and protect your relationships by making it a priority to nurture them.

### Deeper Dive: Technology Reflection

Reflect on how technology and social media impact your life. Consider ways in which they make your life easier or facilitate connection with others. Think about ways in which it may be a distraction. Finally, reflect on how you want to use it intentionally moving forward (e.g. taking time to disconnect).

Here are a few strategies to consider:

1. **Screen time engagement:** If we aren't careful, it's easy to spend most of the day looking at phone, computer, and

television screens. Consider activities you might engage in that will give you a break from screens (for both your eyes and your hands!). Where might you incorporate moments of mindfulness and movement in your day? What can you use to remind you to take breaks? This intentional approach helps maintain focus and promote mental clarity.

2. **Search for wellness apps or tools that support your goals:** For example, meditation apps, habit trackers, and paper or digital planners can help motivate you, structure your day, and track progress toward your goals. What apps or tools might you want to consider adding?

3. **Find what works for you:** There is always going to be a new app or tool that promises to be THE solution for your problems. Remember, advertising is very strategic in calling attention to your problems, but that does not mean that every solution offered is feasible or realistic for you. Pay attention to your lived experience and seek resources that are most beneficial for you. For example, while I do a relatively good job organizing my files, I have yet to find a resource that will effectively help me tackle other digital clutter (e.g., email, photos). This will likely take time, patience, and help, but it is a long-term goal I hope to address.

Remember, technology and social media should *enhance* your life, not detract from it. By conducting a thoughtful audit and implementing boundaries, you can create a digital environment that supports your values and well-being. Embrace these resources as part of your holistic approach to wellness, using them to foster connection, learn new skills, and support your personal growth. Let this be a reminder to use technology wisely, exploring new ways it can bring ease and joy to your life.

## Social Support

Social support is an incredible asset on your wellness journey. Throughout this book, we have discussed the importance of connection with others, finding common humanity, and extending compassion to one another. Asking for help is difficult—it may make you feel vulnerable, there may be cultural norms that associate it with weakness or disrespect, and frankly, some relationships don't feel safe.

But we don't do anything of substance by ourselves.

We rely on the communities we live in to obtain safe sources of food, water, shelter, and social services. We rely on trust in one another as we navigate our daily lives.

When we insist on going it alone, we miss out on the insight and expertise of others who have similar experiences and resources or care deeply about our success.

To consider sources of social support, use the strategies provided in chapter 6, now considering all tiers of your support squad, including your broader network (third tier). Think about who might have useful insights in a particular area of wellness or could serve as an accountability partner.

## Deeper Dive: Social Support Reflection

There are several strategies you can employ to leverage your network effectively:

1. **Take inventory of your existing assets:** Reflect on your existing knowledge or skills and any gaps you would like to address. This will help you make an informed request.
2. **Nurture the relationship:** Ask the other person how you might support them in return. Consider what you have to offer, even if it's as simple as gratitude. Avoid the

mistake of only contacting people when you need their help. Respect their time and appreciate their generosity.

3. **Build a diverse network:** It's valuable to have access to perspectives that help you consider things in a new light. Sometimes, we miss out on people who are helpful because we fail to see what they have to offer. Having several connections helps you avoid a single point of failure. If you rely on one person to be everything to you, losing that relationship will leave you vulnerable.

In the next section, you will begin to build your blueprint. You may find it helpful to refer to the strategies covered in this mini-retreat. Consider which ones resonate with your current needs and circumstances, and how you might want to implement them in your life.

Every step you take to leverage resources in a way that is aligned with your values and priorities is worthy progress.

Be sure to celebrate your wins and ask others for help as needed. Now you'll create a plan that aligns your intentions with meaningful actions for your wellness journey.

MINI-RETREAT #3:
# DESIGN YOUR PATH FORWARD

### Create a Plan That's Authentically Yours

Why do we need a blueprint? Won't we remember everything we've learned and apply it perfectly moving forward?

Yeah, me neither.

We need to be intentional about our wellness because life is unpredictable. We cannot manipulate reality to accommodate all of the promises we've made to ourselves throughout this book.

But when you put in the effort to maintain your practices, you increase your capacity to deal with challenges and build a fulfilling, meaningful life.

You savor positive emotions and seek out sources of awe and joy because you know they provide a counternarrative to the negativity of the world. They help you retain perspective and embrace a growth mindset. This fosters resilience, which fuels resistance, helping you withstand the pressures you face today and a lifetime of tomorrows.

You seek connection and nurture meaningful relationships because you know that we are stronger together than alone.

And you're going to put all this in motion by creating your blueprint for shame-free wellness. As you work on it, remember that there is no one-size-fits-all approach. This blueprint is yours and yours alone. I encourage you to use your journal as you work through this section or go to my website (PortiaPreston.com) for resources that will help you organize your blueprint.

## The SANE Cycle

This blueprint aims to help you create a personalized approach to wellness that you can adapt as your life evolves.

S: Slow down to reflect

A: Acknowledge your current reality

N: Navigate forward with intention

E: Evaluate and adapt

### Step 1: Slow Down to Reflect

First, reflect on what you have learned about your needs and patterns through the mini-retreats in each chapter so far. You may use the following prompts to reflect on each area of wellness. Feel free to modify them to suit your needs.

199

| Area of Wellness | Hustle, Flow, or Let It Go? |
|---|---|
| **Spiritual** | What negatively impacts my sense of worth or my connection to myself, others, or the world around me?<br>Which spiritual practices support my wellness?<br>What do I need to let go of to practice spirituality authentically? |
| **Cognitive** | What makes it difficult for me to think, learn, or process information? How does this impact how I navigate tasks?<br>What systems, tools, or strategies support my executive function?<br>What do I need to let go of to better support my brain's unique needs? |
| **Emotional** | What makes it difficult to honor my authentic emotions or get the support I need?<br>What helps me experience and savor positive emotions? What emotional intelligence skills help me better manage my emotions?<br>What do I need to let go of to better support my emotional needs? |
| **Physical** | What makes it difficult for me to accept my body or tend to my physical needs?<br>What helps me accept and care for my body? Which practices are sustainable for me?<br>What do I need to let go of to foster body compassion and overall physical well-being? |
| **Social** | In what ways do I experience isolation or unhealthy or unsupportive relationships?<br>How can I cultivate a support squad that fulfills my needs?<br>What communication skills or boundaries are helpful in nurturing my relationships?<br>What relationships do I need to let go of? |

| Area of Wellness | Hustle, Flow, or Let It Go? |
|---|---|
| Sense of Self and Roles | What compromises my sense of self outside of what I do? What contributes to burnout in my roles?<br><br>What passions would I like to nurture for myself? What practices help foster well-being in my roles?<br><br>What practices or roles do I need to change my approach to or let go of in order to protect my well-being? |

This reflection will provide you with a baseline to refer to in the future, helping you understand where your needs have changed.

### Step 2: Acknowledge Your Current Reality

Now, it's time to meet yourself right where you are. Start by noting how you feel in this moment. If you feel disconnected from yourself, you can try to establish connection by engaging your senses, using grounding practices like the body scan or sensory scavenger hunt we explored in chapter 5. If you experience discomfort, prioritize establishing a sense of safety.

Consider the following prompts as they are relevant for you. You might choose to focus on a specific topic (e.g. an area of wellness, relationship, role, or responsibility).

| Wellness | Define what wellness means for you through the lens of your experiences. |
|---|---|
| Energy | Explore what might be compromising your energy. |
| Intentions | Note your current priorities and how they are aligned with your values. |

| Time | Reflect on how you protect time for your priorities. Acknowledge what is not under your control. |
|---|---|
| Environment | Consider what elements of your environment support your needs. Note any barriers you face. |
| Finances | Identify your financial priorities and any constraints. |
| Other | Explore other resources (e.g., social support, technology) that can help you address your needs. Note areas in which you face challenges. |

I use these prompts as part of my weekly check-in before creating my schedule. It helps me gain deeper insight into my needs and reality. You can do this independently or discuss it with a trusted friend or your loved ones.

If you would like to capture your current wellness needs and compare them to your blueprint in step 1, consider the following prompts:

| Spiritual | Contemplate your sense of self-worth, connection to something greater than yourself, or other spiritual needs. |
|---|---|
| Cognitive | Note your thought patterns without judging them. Identify assumptions or beliefs that might not be rooted in reality. |
| Emotional | Assess your current emotional state. |
| Physical | Reflect on your relationship with your body and your needs for nourishment, rest, movement, and care. |

| | |
|---|---|
| **Social** | Explore your needs for meaningful connection and where you are experiencing difficulties with communication or boundaries. |
| **Sense of Self and Roles** | Consider how you can nurture your passions outside of your roles. Identify factors that support or compromise your well-being in your roles and responsibilities. |

These small actions can help you gain clarity about your next steps. Remember to be compassionate with yourself as you assess your needs, refraining from judgment. If you are experiencing shame in any of these areas, refer to the sidebar titled "Step Out of the Shame Spiral" for help.

### Step 3: Navigate Forward with Intention

You are now ready to create an action plan that is anchored in your reality. Consider the following steps:

| | |
|---|---|
| **Desired Outcome** | Define what you hope to achieve and why it matters to you. |
| **Approach** | Brainstorm options that are realistic and aligned with your values. |
| **Process** | Set meaningful and measurable milestones. Identify small, doable steps that are clearly defined. Troubleshoot potential roadblocks. Implement systems where possible. |
| **Resources** | Consider your strengths, skills, and knowledge, as well as any resources you can leverage. In what ways might you benefit from accountability? |
| **Wellness Practices** | Incorporate relevant practices to protect your capacity and foster resilience. |

## Step Out of the Shame Spiral[4]

We begin by bringing experiences of unhealthy shame into the light. Shame thrives in silence, often lurking in the corners of our lives. We conceal our flaws, fearing exposure and judgment. But addressing shame head-on is a mindset move that can transform your life.

1. **Recognize the trigger:** Shame can start as a slow simmer, a whisper of doubt, or a feeling that you should be farther along than you are. Or it can come on suddenly, perhaps triggered by a mistake you made or an external event like rejection or unexpected criticism. Before you know it, you're stuck. It's important to know that while it feels real, it does not reflect the truth of who you are.

2. **Connect with yourself:** Engage your senses to reconnect with the present moment. Focus on what is easily accessible: what you can see, hear, feel, smell, or taste. These small actions can help you regain control of your energy and attention, helping you find clarity on how to move forward.

3. **Be curious:** Beware of the shame sinkhole. This is where you feel stuck, and with no other way out, you sink deeper into shame. No matter how long you ruminate on what you or someone else could or should have done, playing the blame game will never edit your reality. It will only dig you a deeper hole.

   What might you do instead? Focus on a small action that is doable in this moment and represents a small step forward. If you feel safe exploring your body's response, try rating the intensity of the sensations you feel on a scale of 1 (lowest) to 10 (highest). Explore what is helpful to you—perhaps it's deep breaths, taking a break, or noting your thoughts and emotions, all without judgment. You might reflect on how you have handled a similar situation in the past.

Note: Sometimes we don't have the energy to care for ourselves or notice our needs. In these moments, we need safety and connection. Find someone who is supportive and understanding—a friend with whom you have built trust or a professional. Vulnerability (in the right hands) is not a weakness but a bridge to deeper connection.

4. **Reflect:** Once the spiral has passed and you feel safe, reflect on your experience. What did you learn? What insights might you use to help you in the future? What might you want to do differently, and what support do you need to take that step? Let curiosity transform challenges into opportunities for growth.

Dealing with shame is not a linear journey. This is an ongoing practice, and you will learn over time what approaches work best for you. Feel free to modify this and make it your own.

### Step 4: Evaluate and Adapt

You can assess your progress toward milestones at regular intervals (e.g., weekly, monthly, quarterly). Here are a few prompts you could use:

Celebrate wins, large or small.

Reflect on setbacks and lessons learned.

Determine where to adapt your approach or let go.

Regular check-ins ensure you are responsive to your evolving reality.

You might also consider using assessments to identify and address emergent wellness needs. For example, I find it helpful to take the PERMAH survey* on a quarterly basis to assess how my professional role is impacting my overall well-being.

Set regular appointments to evaluate your ongoing needs and resources. Here are a few examples:

1. **Review upcoming commitments:** Note where you may be committed beyond your capacity. Consider what you might be able to delegate, postpone, or eliminate.

2. **Reconcile finances:** Review your spending patterns and adjust your budget as needed.

3. **Assess your environment:** Evaluate your needs in your home, workplace, and public spaces. Consider what strategies, tools, or support might be helpful in caring for your needs.

4. **Stay on top of your health care needs:** Keep up with scheduled screenings and access care to address emerging or ongoing health needs.

These check-ins can help you troubleshoot and address issues before they spiral out of control. As you become more familiar with your needs and patterns, you will be able to better identify strategies and systems that work for you. Your plan is here to serve you. Approach it from a place of connection with your needs and reality, not perfection.

## Flow Menu: Rolling with Reality

There is power in flexibility. A flow menu provides options for wellness practices based on your interests, energy, and available resources.

---

*This survey examines well-being in a workplace context in six areas: positive emotions, engagement, relationships, meaning, accomplishment, and health.

Consider what you might do on each of the following types of days:

1. **Slow days:** When you are low on time or energy, focus on simple efforts that nurture your well-being, such as breathing exercises, short walks, or meditation breaks.
2. **Steady days:** This is your baseline routine for ongoing maintenance. Here, the aim is to maintain consistency by focusing on activities that are feasible for your daily life. If you crave variety like I do, try to give yourself a few options.
3. **Stretch days:** On these days, you have the capacity to challenge yourself or try something new. Consider options that will foster growth and develop your personal or professional skillsets.

Stay attuned to how you're feeling and adjust your approach as needed.

## Emergency Self-Care Plan

We should *always* have a plan for challenging times. I strongly suggest both making a plan for yourself as outlined below and sharing this with a trusted member of your support squad who could help you implement this plan if needed.

1. **Set the environment:** Explore what makes you feel calm (e.g., music, scents, candles, quiet).
2. **Meet your basic needs:** Consider supportive strategies to ensure you are able to eat, hydrate, and rest. On my most difficult days, I turn my to-do list into a "grace list." I focus only on the things I must do to get through the day.
3. **Cope with stress:** Identify practices that help you restore a sense of calm or be present in the moment. Make sure

they are easy to access when you need them. This might include your favorite guided meditations, a breathwork or yoga practice, or stretches that help you relax.

4. **Tap into your support squad:** Consider which members of your squad (or trusted professionals) you can contact if you need support. Consider communicating ahead of time what type of support you might find helpful in the case of an emergency.

This plan can help you find easily accessible ways to care for yourself during difficult times.

---

You did it! You tackled a first draft of your wellness blueprint based on where you are today. You can feel free to return to this and modify it as needed. However, you have a plan in place, and that is worthy of celebration.

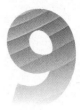

# Wellness Beyond Ourselves

*A Vision for the Collective*

Take a moment to recall all that you have explored on this journey, and what these experiences have served to affirm:

- Your inherent worth and the restoration of connection to yourself, others, and the world around you
- The unique needs of your brain
- The validity of your full range of emotions
- The nourishment of your body and care for its needs
- Connection with a supportive community
- A strong sense of self outside of what you do for others and protection from burnout in your roles and responsibilities

You now have tools that will help you identify sustainable wellness practices that will support you in each season of your life as you navigate challenges and uncertainty.

Maybe you've heard of the slow movement. This philosophy, introduced by Carl Honoré, is not about doing everything slowly but about finding the "right speed" by being aware of what is required in balance with our priorities.[1] Likewise, an ongoing practice to navigate the hustle, find flow, and let go requires nuance.

Most of us cannot completely eliminate the hustle from our lives. It's in our culture, and for many, it's part of our roles and responsibilities. Also, some people enjoy the thrill of the hustle. But we have to stay alert for when the hustle begins to have a negative impact on our lives, and be ready to adapt using the skills we have discussed throughout this book.

The practices that help us cultivate flow in one season will likely need to be adjusted as we move to another. Also, there will always be some factors that inhibit flow, whether it's resistance, internalized messages, or the impacts of systems on our lives. We have to be agile in order to shift with our needs and reality.

Finally, letting go can be complicated. If you are letting go of a task, role, or relationship that has held a significant place in your life, it can feel devastating. And letting go is not always our choice. We may need time to grieve and recover.

As we move through seasons of life, it may also seem like the problems we face are increasingly difficult. We might wonder if it's worth continuing to put ourselves out there and take risks. The chances of failure or rejection can increase as we challenge ourselves to stretch toward higher goals.

One thing that helps me discern if I am truly invested in a new opportunity is to ask myself if it is worth the risk of rejection. Then, I visualize what is possible if I face my fears and overcome them, rather than allowing them to stare me down. I might remind myself that even if I experience defeat, it is not an indictment of who I am. I am still worthy. Keeping this at the front of my mind helps motivate me to take the time I need to heal, seek out support, and look for ways to pivot forward.

The mini-retreats in this chapter are designed to prepare you for future challenges and opportunities. You will explore how to face the prospect of letting go with courage. You will also consider ways to contribute to the well-being of others you interact with where you live, work, play, and serve.

In the powerful words of bell hooks, "I contemplate what our lives would be like if we knew how to cultivate awareness, to live mindfully, peacefully; if we learned habits of being that would bring us closer together, that would help us build beloved community."[2] This work you've done in yourself is *important*. And it can produce a ripple effect on the greater sea of humanity, bringing us one step closer to collective wellness.

## RETREAT RESET

Imagine standing before a large pond filled with lotus flowers. Here, you're invited to reflect on the journey of the lotus—revered across many cultures, this flower is a symbol for purity, resilience, and enlightenment.

While celebrated for its beautiful blossom, this is only a small part of its life. The lotus begins as a seed, lying dormant for years until the right conditions arise. Perhaps blown by the wind into a body of water, it settles into the mud at the bottom—an unlikely origin for most plant life. From here, it grows strong roots capable of drawing nourishment from the murky depths.

It takes a year for the stem and leaves to reach the surface, and then they form a protective boundary that allows the lotus to blossom in the second year. For about five days, it shines gloriously. During this brief window, its goal is to pollinate, releasing seeds to begin the cycle anew.

This journey serves as a metaphor for our own. Just as it's not guaranteed that a seed will find the right conditions to grow, not everything we attempt will succeed. It's unrealistic to expect we'll never experience failure—it's a part of life.

It's crucial that we don't define ourselves by our struggles. If we do, we'll miss out on the fullness of our life journey. Instead, we must make an ongoing commitment to stay rooted and connected, creating practices that help stabilize our foundation. Just as the lotus's stem and leaves ensure the flower's safety, you must use boundaries to protect what you value.

MINI-RETREAT #1:

## MOVE BEYOND INDIVIDUALISM

### Finding the Intersection of Your Well-Being and the Collective

Now that we have learned the lessons of wellness at an individual level, how do we scale what we have learned to impact others?

One of the major criticisms of wellness is that too much focus is placed on the individual. This is not where our journey should end.

For example, self-compassion should strengthen our ability to be kind to others, helping us better understand their experiences and find common ground. We can become more observant of how others are being treated and aim to act in alignment with our values to address harm and protect each other.

Inclusive wellness considers the needs of all. It starts with the individual but extends to the collective. It involves expanding our awareness beyond ourselves and those with whom we have relationships to understand that we are part of a greater whole.

We all have a vested interest in strengthening the collective, as it ultimately impacts our own wellness. Consider how the metaphor of putting on your own oxygen mask before helping others with theirs might apply in this context.

As a baseline, everyone deserves clean air.

We rely on systems to ensure the air is free of pollutants and that the masks are functioning properly.

Once we have secured our own oxygen mask, we have a collective responsibility to ensure others are able to breathe as well.

Without collective wellness, individual wellness is a fallacy. Collective wellness is forged across multiple levels. Interpersonal relationships provide accountability and opportunities to engage in communal care, while efforts we engage in within organizations or at the community level are essential for securing needed resources and advocating for policies that support needs of whole populations. This can include access to affordable housing, clean water, quality food, health care, and safe parks and trails.

The African humanist philosophy of Ubuntu defines humanity as the expression of our interconnectedness through relationship, generosity, and kindness. Consider the contrast between how our society defines success and this perspective offered by Archbishop Desmond Tutu: "When you have this quality—Ubuntu—you are known for your generosity. We think of ourselves far too frequently as just individuals, separated from one another, whereas you are connected and what you do affects the whole world. When you do well, it spreads out; it is for the whole of humanity."[3]

## REFLECTION

Explore how your wellness journey is impacted by the collective and how you can impact others.

1. **Individual:** What factors promote or hinder my wellness and that of others in my community?
2. **Interpersonal relationships:** What role, if any, does my connection to others (peers, family, colleagues) play in my wellness? How might I influence their wellness?
3. **Communities:** How do the available resources and the environment I live in (e.g., safe drinking water, facilities for exercise) shape my wellness and that of others in my community?
4. **Organizations:** How do the settings in which I carry out daily activities (e.g., schools, workplaces, churches)

influence my wellness? How can I partner with individuals or organizations in my community to promote collective wellness (extending beyond myself)?

5. **Societal norms and policies:** How do the policies or norms (practices that are accepted as normal) in my society (local, state, federal) influence my wellness? How do systemic barriers (e.g., the absence of a livable wage) work against wellness?

Think of the ripple effect we can have in the communities we serve as we embody the courage to slow down and reflect on our practices.

## MINI-RETREAT #2:
# CREATE YOUR VISION FOR THE COLLECTIVE

### Addressing Wellness on Multiple Levels

What would you include in your vision for collective wellness? For example, you might envision a world in which we all have what we need and treat each other with compassion and dignity. Think about some of the values that are important to you in the context of community, such as inclusion, belonging, safety, or equity. You might reflect on aspects of the hustle that impact your own journey and the lives of others to help you determine what is important to you, such as providing access to resources, freedom from discrimination, and protection from harm.

I encourage you to start at the local level by considering those you interact with daily. How can you affirm their worth and support their journey? Start by nurturing strong connections with trust, so that there is a foundation of safety. If people are willing to share their struggles, listen as you have capacity. If you have relevant experiences, offer to share them to the extent you feel safe doing so. This may help foster common humanity. As you process your own narrative, you may already be thinking about how you can help others. Before you reach out to someone and say, "Hey, I found this really great strategy that you should try! This will work for you!" it's important to take a moment to process the journey that brought you to this point.

Be mindful that it was shaped by several factors unique to your life. For example, what was going on in your life before you picked up this book? What compelled you to keep reading? (Thank you, by the way!) While information is powerful, the tips in this book are not enough by themselves to motivate you to take steps forward. Events in your life, your access to resources, influential relationships that reinforce your decisions, and your core values are other factors that may play a large role in compelling you to make a change.

Think for a moment about the position of the people you wish to share your journey with, whether they are your loved ones, colleagues, or part of your extended community. Even if the same events were to happen to them, it is likely that they have their own unique response.

It is important to respect the autonomy of others to navigate their own journey and to have different goals.

Reflect on the work you have done to develop compassion for yourself, especially in the areas in which you struggle. Sit with this for a moment. Remember, the confidence you are now developing in areas of wellness might have been timidity or avoidance not long ago.

Take a deep breath.

Perhaps you had an epiphany about caring for your body in a way that is authentic for you, or you have decided you are ready to go to therapy. You might look at someone else and think, *Wow, they have the same issues I do! I can help them get help too!*

Stop.

Even if you are close, you don't know their journey. I'm confident about this because sometimes my *own* journey is a mystery to me. You don't know what points might be triggering for them, or perhaps there are things you can see that they are not yet aware of. You can do emotional harm by forcing the conversation when they are not ready. It is not your job to reveal other people's trauma to them or force them to work through it. It's possible they do not desire help or that they need to get that help from someone else. Be careful to honor other people's boundaries and resist the belief that you know what is best for them.

Now let's think about how you can be supportive in relationships in your life. The most important step is to think about how you can model compassion for other people. And that starts with having compassion for yourself. Be mindful of where they are in their life right now. Think about the fact that we cycle back and forth between addressing our need for growth and our need for safety. This will help you be gentler with your conversation. Don't assume that they are at a point where they are ready to make this change. Think about how we all have different needs, preferences, levels of exposure to stress, and ways of coping.

You can share in a way that does not create pressure by speaking to the journey that you are on without being attached to how they respond. Remember, you can be proud of the steps you are taking to be more vulnerable, to extend compassion to yourself, and to intentionally engage in deep care, without needing someone else to validate your experience. It's natural for our ego to want everyone around us to get on board. Have compassion for this feeling. Developing this sensitivity will help you be respectful of other people.

## Be Mindful of Your Capacity

If you know someone who is going through a challenging situation, think about realistic and tangible ways that you could offer support without straining yourself. For example, if I wanted to be supportive of a friend who wants to start being more physically active, I might offer to check in with them via text to provide accountability. Or I could meet up with them occasionally for a walk. However, I am not open to meeting them at the gym in their neighborhood at four o'clock in the morning! That does not honor my capacity regarding my available time or energy. You can be creative in thinking about ways to support others while being mindful of your boundaries.

I have another example from when I was planning to undergo my hysterectomy. I was mindful of how often I felt alone going through this process. While I knew many women who dealt with fibroids, most were exploring alternative options that would preserve their fertility. I decided that once I had undergone my procedure, I would find a way to capture my narrative for others to have as a resource in the future. I decided to create a series of videos about my experience that captured my recovery for six months post-surgery. I protected my privacy by only speaking about the procedure once it was complete and I was at home resting. I also protected ethical boundaries by refusing to counsel others on what is a highly personal decision.

Now, consider how you might impact others through your roles. Here is an example of how leaders in the workplace might approach this.

Leaders play an influential role in promoting a culture of wellness in the workplace. They can help create an environment that promotes psychological safety by welcoming questions, seeing mistakes as an opportunity for learning and growth rather than shame, and encouraging individuals to take risks that can help move the organization forward. They can provide opportunities for people to share anonymously how policies and practices might be contributing to burnout, and follow through with responsive action.

If a leader is in a field where employees provide direct support to clients who may have experienced trauma, they can take steps to address the emotional burden of the work, ensuring that they are prepared to recognize the signs of secondary traumatic stress and burnout. Leaders can also help combat incivility in the workplace culture by encouraging compassion, which is a proactive step against bullying and other tactics that diminish psychological safety.

Furthermore, leaders can prioritize creating space for others to care for themselves, authentically engage in such spaces, and regularly encourage employees to use their time to take advantage of available resources. Many organizations have an employee assistance program that goes underutilized by employees because either they are not aware that it is available, they've had a prior negative experience that has decreased their faith in its ability to help them, or they don't have time to take advantage of the available resources.

Leaders should give thought on a regular basis to how they are prioritizing work, as scope creep typically falls on the shoulders of employees who are not in a position to set boundaries or delegate. They should think about possible alterations to the way work is managed or organized to ensure a more reasonable workload. Trainings that simply educate people on topics such as burnout or stressors such as racism do not go far enough. Trainings that identify root causes, equip people with effective tools, and inform action can be helpful, if paired with structural change and accountability.

Whether or not we are all leaders, we all have the power to advocate in our own ways (even if we are introverted and need to find quiet ways to do so!). We have the capacity to shape social norms and inform policy at the local, state, and national level. To do this, it's important to think about the experiences that we've discussed in this book through an intersectional lens, understanding that the more marginalized an identity someone occupies, the more compounded the effect on their wellness. For example, someone who does not have access to mental health services, food, shelter, and other resources that foster wellness will have additional struggles compared to someone of a similar background who has a stable income or an adequate income.

### REFLECTION

Consider how you can contribute to collective wellness from your position:

1. Think of tangible ways in which you can positively impact others, such as treating people with respect and compassion in daily interactions.
2. Think about how you might influence others in your role, family, workplace, or community.
3. Consider how you might advocate for change to address systemic issues and engage in collective action to realize well-being for all.

MINI-RETREAT #3:

## HARNESS YOUR INDIVIDUAL JOURNEY TO IMPACT COLLECTIVE WELLNESS

### Putting What You Have Learned into Practice

Shortly after my adviser's passing, I house-sat for her wife on several occasions. One day, I decided to take a morning walk to a beautiful outdoor mall. On my walk home, I had just crossed the intersection when I noticed an older Asian man walking toward me. He jumped off the sidewalk and into the street and began screaming the N-word at the top of his lungs, over and over again, careful to stay as far away from me as possible.

I was not nearly as shocked by his behavior as by what happened next.

Despite being surrounded by people on the sidewalk, no one said a word to intervene, nor to check on me afterward. I'm confident they went home that day and told stories about the interaction, exclaiming to their loved ones, "You're not going to believe what happened when I went out today!"

In that moment, I had to pull myself together and continue walking alone. In an act of what had to be divine providence, one block later I was approached by a Black man with dreadlocks. He looked politely in my direction, saying, "Beautiful," and continued on his way. While this did help in the moment, the shock I felt from the incident stayed with me for years.

It has taken some deep inner work to reflect on the verbal assault, recalling that the man screamed as if he were in deep pain. If my mere presence was enough to set him off and compel him to seek safety in traffic, what might he have been dealing with inside? While I did not know the source of that pain, I knew he absorbed or learned it in a context that had nothing to do with me. Growing up in South Central Los Angeles, I was not naive to the tensions that existed between Black and Asian communities. I was used to the mistrust when I entered shops, feeling as if my every move was monitored with a lingering, suspicious stare.

However, I had also known many people who were kind, and I had grown up with close friends with family roots in China, Vietnam, and Korea. I was woefully unprepared for such a heinous act of ignorance and hatred. I was naive in the sense that I could not imagine a community could simultaneously consist of individuals who are committed to reconciliation and healing and those who have doubled down on their pain, allowing it to fester and metastasize.

I could have chosen to respond by allowing this incident to form a narrative that spoke for all, ultimately consuming me.

Instead, I chose to breathe slowly, feeling the pain. It would continue to ripple in my heart for years. I envisioned some type of community that could help me process this and put it into context, but I didn't know who to reach out to. I discussed it occasionally, mostly when helping friends or students process similar events that had happened to them. Several years later, early in the Covid-19 pandemic, our department decided to take a public stand against anti-Asian hate. In working with close friends from the Asian community, I took a chance and allowed myself to be vulnerable, sharing my experience.

My friend listened deeply, acknowledging my pain. When I asked for insight on the pain of elders in her community, she offered her perspective without making any excuses. What we shared deepened our bond with each other and our commitment to advancing healing in both of our communities.

I still return to think about this incident sometimes, because a remnant of pain does linger. I think about the layers of that moment, how it pointed to moments from earlier in life I had not processed. What I know now is that the narrative that formed in that man's heart impacted me. The reluctance of bystanders to check on me, even after the moment passed, wounded my belief in common humanity. However, I ultimately healed in community, both with those who shared my identity and had similar experiences and those who acknowledged the source of the inflicted pain within their own communities.

I found that the love of a community is a balm for hatred that illuminates a collective path forward.

You might find yourself wondering, *Is collective healing even possible? How can we come together in a world that is increasingly divisive?*

We must contend with what came before us—the effects of war, migration, genocide, the Holocaust, and slavery. These atrocities have wounded our humanity, leaving as their legacy systems that perpetuate supremacy, drive inequity, and leave intergenerational scars.

It can be overwhelming to face the challenge of using what we have to build something better, restoring connection and equity where division has taken root. This work cannot be done alone; we need each other. We ignore the call to restore our humanity at our own peril. We have to combat a narrative that justifies division based on who we are, where we come from, or what we have.

Our humanity is not bound only by spirit but by blood. We are not as different as societal narratives or political rhetoric may lead us to believe.

For example, it is nearly impossible for many descendants of enslaved people and slaveowners to disentangle their ancestry. Consider the connection between Motown founder Berry Gordy III and President Jimmy Carter. In 1978, Berry Gordy III's family discovered they shared ancestry with President Carter, tracing their roots back to James Thomas Gordy, a plantation owner in Georgia. President Carter's lineage came from Gordy's children with his wife, while Berry Gordy III descended from Berry Gordy, the child of an enslaved woman named Ester Johnson.[4]

In our current era, we are increasingly prone to calling out those who have done harm. However, healing rarely occurs by cutting ourselves off from those who have caused damage. If we have not healed the source of the wound, it will only manifest in new ways. How do we correct our course? We must create a better world, one in which inclusion can thrive. We must walk our talk outside of the workplace and the classroom and into every area of our lives.

These stories show us that there is more that unites us than divides us. Recognizing this truth affirms our shared humanity and emphasizes the importance of addressing old wounds. Healing rather than suppressing is essential.

We must learn to communicate across differences and recognize the humanity in each other. By moving past rigid perspectives and rejecting false superiority, we can foster a more united and compassionate world.

## REFLECTION

1. What lessons have you learned on your own journey that have taught you the importance of inclusion?
2. How can we embrace inclusion when division feels safer?
3. What steps have you taken, or do you want to take, to connect more deeply with others who are different from you?

## An Inclusive Approach to Wellness

I continue to explore my own role in collective healing. The work I do across sectors helps leaders create organizational cultures that promote well-being. We start with assessing the well-being of the individual in the context of the workplace using indicators of flourishing: positive emotions, engagement, relationships, meaning, accomplishment, and health.

We then tie in the principles discussed throughout this book to foster collective wellness. For example, self-awareness and mindful self-compassion can help improve respect and cohesion, combatting shame and incivility. Improving skills related to emotional and social intelligence can help foster psychological safety, making it safer to ask for help, lead with transparency, and take the risks required for innovation. With this foundation, teams can leverage each other's strengths and overcome obstacles to solve pressing problems in our world.

Now, think about your own life. How can you put your vision for collective wellness into practice by using your own healing journey to help others, and letting other people's journeys inform yours?

We are strongest when we are united in our humanity—seeing ourselves in each other and accepting that our fates are interwoven. Like Fred Rogers says, "The world needs a sense of worth, and it will achieve it only by its people feeling that they are worthwhile."[5]

From this standpoint, we can be effective allies for each other. Together, we can ride the waves of life with more awareness, presence, compassion, and intention, proactively addressing critical needs in our society.

You're not here to fix yourself or anyone else. You are here to love.

You love yourself with each step you take toward healing, accepting your worth, meeting your needs, and evolving into the fullest, most authentic expression of yourself.

We love each other by showing compassion, listening to understand, celebrating what makes us unique, and employing our talents, skills, and resources in service of the greater good. Each of these are portals of connection that allow us to tap into the strength of our shared humanity.

Our humanity is our greatest asset, creating the foundation for a collective pursuit of wellness that benefits us all.

# One Final Note

It is my hope that sharing my experiences brings a sense of common humanity to all who are navigating life's challenges. I know my words would not have flowed with as much grace and vulnerability, nor would my story have been as resonant or compelling, had my journey been easy or straightforward.

As you revisit this book in the years to come (and I truly hope you do!), you may find that while you have evolved and established more flow in some areas of wellness, others continue to be impacted by the hustle. Some of the things you let go of might reappear in new forms. This is the nature of life. The key is to meet yourself where you are.

Every day offers a new opportunity to choose:

To let go of the quest for control and perfection
To embrace presence, love, and connection
To care for ourselves
To care for humanity

Choose wisely.

May this book accompany you through new seasons, bringing fresh insights and a hopeful perspective to the horizon ahead.

# Acknowledgments

The journey of this book, birthed from an unexpected vision at the age of nineteen, has led me to connect with myself, cultivate safety, and release shame—transforming how I see myself and my purpose. As it comes to an end, it has taken on new meaning. It has become a love letter to humanity.

My family's love and unwavering belief in me have allowed my dreams to sustain flight. To my husband, thank you for a love that transcends words; you are a lifetime of answered prayers. I am grateful to my mother, who nurtured my abilities with her unique recipe for success: opportunity, sacrifice, support, patience, and integrity. Thank you to my father, who has been a constant source of encouragement and support. To my brother, I realize now our "twin sense" was a shared brilliance. Growing up feeling different wasn't easy, but I'm grateful I didn't have to do it alone.

With profound gratitude, I honor my extended family and ancestral lineages—Vernon, Dyson, Reed, Hopson, and Morris. I carry their strength, wisdom, and teachings within me.

Thank you to my editors at Revell who championed this project from start to finish. To my writing coaches and literary friends, thank you for helping my thoughts find written expression.

I am grateful to my community at Cal State Fullerton and Cal State LA for their steadfast encouragement of my journey. To my students, clients, and audiences, your courage and vulnerability breathed inspiration into each page.

To my friends, my own constellation of stars, you always make me feel seen, loved, valued, and understood just as I am. Thank you for listening to a thousand different versions of this story and, before that, letting me beta test free advice for years as I honed my craft. I hope you know how much you have taught me. I am in awe that I get to do life with you.

I am grateful for the many spaces that have provided me with a respite from the world over the years. And to you, dear reader: May your own experiences with retreats in this book and beyond be an ongoing invitation to surrender to ease.

# Notes

### A Letter to the Reader

1. George Plimpton, "Maya Angelou, The Art of Fiction No. 119," *Paris Review*, 1990, accessed October 2, 2024, https://www.theparisreview.org/interviews/2279/the-art-of-fiction-no-119-maya-angelou.

2. Plimpton, "Maya Angelou."

### Introduction

1. American Association of University Women, "Systemic Racism and the Gender Pay Gap: A Supplement to The Simple Truth," 2021, https://www.aauw.org/app/uploads/2021/07/SimpleTruth_4.0-1.pdf. The pay gap refers to differences in pay between population groups, and points to a history of undervaluing labor that continues today. In 2019–20, for every dollar earned by a White man, Asian women earned 87 cents, White women earned 79 cents, Black women and Native Hawaiian and Other Pacific Islander women earned 63 cents, American Indian and Alaskan Native women earned 60 cents, and Hispanic/Latinx women earned 55 cents.

2. Mathilde Roux, "5 Facts About Black Women in the Labor Force," *U.S. Department of Labor Blog*, August 3, 2021, https://blog.dol.gov/2021/08/03/5-facts-about-black-women-in-the-labor-force.

3. Malissa Clark et al., "All Work and No Play? A Meta-Analytic Examination of the Correlates and Outcomes of Workaholism," *Journal of Management* 42, no. 7 (2016): 1836–73.

4. R. N. Carleton, M. K. Mulvogue, and S. Duranceau, "PTSD Personality Subtypes in Women Exposed to Intimate-Partner Violence," *Psychological Trauma: Theory, Research, Practice, and Policy* 7, no. 2 (2015): 154–61, https://doi.org/10.1037/tra0000003.

5. Z. Chouliara, T. Karatzias, and A. Gullone, "Recovering from Childhood Sexual Abuse: A Theoretical Framework for Practice and Research," *Journal of Psychiatric and Mental Health Nursing* 21, no. 1 (2014): 69–78.

6. Cecilie Schou Andreassen et al., "The Relationships Between Workaholism and Symptoms of Psychiatric Disorders: A Large-Scale Cross-Sectional Study," *PLOS ONE* 11, no. 5 (2016), https://doi.org/10.1371/journal.pone.0152978.

7. Tanya Paperny, "Do Some Trauma Survivors Cope by Overworking?," *Atlantic*, February 16, 2017, https://www.theatlantic.com/health/archive/2017/02/do-some-trauma-survivors-cope-by-overworking/516540/.

8. Cheryl L. Woods-Giscombé, "Superwoman Schema: African American Women's Views on Stress, Strength, and Health," *Qualitative Health Research* 20.5 (2010): 668–83.

9. Portia Jackson Preston et al., "Serving Students Takes a Toll: Self-Care, Health, and Professional Quality of Life," *Journal of Student Affairs Research and Practice* 58, no. 2 (2021): 163–78.

10. Jackson Preston et al., "Serving Students."

## Chapter 1 Cultivating Self-Awareness

1. Jeff Foster Live, accessed November 6, 2024, www.jefffosteronline.com.

2. Arline T. Geronimus et al., "Do US Black Women Experience Stress-Related Accelerated Biological Aging?: A Novel Theory and First Population-Based Test of Black-White Differences in Telomere Length," *Human Nature* 21 (2010): 19–38, https://doi.org/10.1007/s12110-010-9078-0.

## Chapter 2 Accepting Your Intrinsic Worth

1. John Fisher, "The Four Domains Model: Connecting Spirituality, Health, and Well-Being," *Religions* 2, no. 1 (2011): 17–28.

2. Toni Morrison, *Beloved* (Vintage, 2007), 273.

3. "The 24 Character Strengths," VIA Institute on Character, accessed November 10, 2024, https://www.viacharacter.org/character-strengths.

## Chapter 3 Exploring Your Thoughts

1. Kristin D. Neff, "The Development and Validation of a Scale to Measure Self-Compassion," *Self and Identity* 2, no. 3 (2003): 223–50.

2. Russell Barkley, "What Is Executive Function? 7 Deficits Tied to ADHD," *ADDitude Magazine*, updated October 13, 2019, https://www.additudemag.com/7-executive-function-deficits-linked-to-adhd/.

3. "Executive Dysfunction," Cleveland Clinic, updated June 5, 2022, https://my.clevelandclinic.org/health/symptoms/23224-executive-dysfunction.

4. Christina Metcalf et al., "Cognitive Problems in Perimenopause: A Review of Recent Evidence," *Current Psychiatry Reports* 25, no. 10 (2023): 501–11, https://doi.org/10.1007/s11920-023-01447-3.

5. Elisabeth Nordenswan et al.,"Maternal Psychological Distress and Executive Functions Are Associated During Early Parenthood—A FinnBrain Birth Cohort Study," *Frontiers in Psychology* 12 (2021), https://doi.org/10.3389/fpsyg.2021.719996.

6. Audreyana Jagger-Rickels et al., "An Executive Function Subtype of PTSD with Unique Neural Markers and Clinical Trajectories," *Translational Psychiatry* 12, no. 262 (2022), https://doi.org/10.1038/s41398-022-02011-y.

7. Gabriel R. Gilmore et al., "Sleep/Wake Regularity Influences How Stress Shapes Executive Function," *Frontiers in Sleep* 3 (2024), https://doi.org/10.3389/frsle.2024.1359723.

8. David D. Burns, "Checklist of Cognitive Distortions," adapted from *Feeling Good: The New Mood Therapy* (William Morrow & Company, 1980).

9. "Key Substance Use and Mental Health Indicators in the United States: Results from the 2022 National Survey on Drug Use and Health," Substance Abuse and Mental Health Services Administration, November 13, 2023, https://www.samhsa.gov/data/report/2022-nsduh-annual-national-report.

10. National Cancer Institute, "Neurodiversity," *Division of Cancer and Epidemiology*, April 25, 2022, https://dceg.cancer.gov/about/diversity-inclusion/inclusivity-minute/2022/neurodiversity.

11. Centers for Disease Control and Prevention, "Promoting Mental Health and Well-Being in Schools," *Division of Adolescent Health*, updated March 22, 2024, https://www.cdc.gov/healthyyouth/mental-health-action-guide/index.html.

12. University of San Diego, "5 Ways Educators Can Support Neurodiversity in the Classroom," *School for Leadership and Education Sciences*, June 5, 2023, https://solesstories.sandiego.edu/degree-of-difference/5-ways-educators-can-support-neurodiversity-in-the-classroom.

13. Jack Kelly, "How to Create a More Inclusive Environment for Neurodivergent Employees," *Forbes Magazine*, July 22, 2024, https://www.forbes.com/sites/jackkelly/2024/07/22/how-to-create-a-more-inclusive-work-environment-for-neurodivergent-employees/.

## Chapter 4 Managing Your Emotions

1. Paul Ekman, "Universals and Cultural Differences in Facial Expressions of Emotions," in *Nebraska Symposium on Motivation*, ed. J. Cole, (University of Nebraska Press, 1972), 207–82.

2. Gloria Wilcox, *The Feeling Wheel*, Positive Psychology Practitioner's Toolkit, https://www.gnyha.org/wp-content/uploads/2020/05/The-Feeling-Wheel-Positive-Psycology-Program.pdf.

3. American Psychological Association, "Stress in America 2022: Concerned for The Future, Beset by Inflation," October 2022, https://www.apa.org/news/press/releases/stress/2022/concerned-future-inflation.

4. Jeanne Marie Laskas, "The Mister Rogers No One Saw," *New York Times*, November 19, 2019, www.nytimes.com/2019/11/19/magazine/mr-rogers.html.

5. Lauri Nummenmaa et al., "Bodily Maps of Emotions," *Proceedings of the National Academy of Sciences* 111, no. 2 (2014): 646–51.

6. Wilcox, *The Feeling Wheel*.

7. Lane Gillespie, "Survey: 47% of Americans Say Money Is Negatively Impacting Their Mental Health," *Bankrate*, May 9, 2024, https://www.bankrate.com/loans/personal-loans/money-and-mental-health-survey/.

8. Multi-Health Systems, Emotional Quotient-Inventory 2.0 Manual (2011), https://cdn.mhs.com/mhsdocs/EQi20Manual/index.html. Based on the original BarOn EQ-1 authored by Rueven Bar-On (1997).

9. Ryan Dunn, "Mr. Rogers' Words for Times of Tragedy," United Methodist Communications, August 7, 2019, https://www.umc.org/en/content/mr-rogers -words-for-times-of-tragedy.

10. Carol S. Dweck, *Mindset: The New Psychology of Success* (Random House, 2006).

11. Christine Gross-Loh, "How Praise Became a Consolation Prize," *The Atlantic*, December 16, 2016, https://www.theatlantic.com/education/archive/2016 /12/how-praise-became-a-consolation-prize/510845/.

## Chapter 5 Flaws and All

1. Jennifer K. Altman et al., "The Body Compassion Scale: Development and Initial Validation," *Journal of Health Psychology* 25, no. 4 (2020): 439–49.

2. Samantha Artiga et al., "Survey on Racism, Discrimination and Health: Experiences and Impacts Across Racial and Ethnic Groups," Kaiser Family Foundation, December 5, 2023, https://www.kff.org/report-section/survey-on-racism -discrimination-and-health-findings/.

3. Yendelela Cuffee et al., "Examining Race-Based and Gender-Based Discrimination, Trust in Providers, and Mental Well-Being Among Black Women," *Journal of Racial and Ethnic Health Disparities* (2024), https://doi.org/10.1007 /s40615-024-01913-5.

## Chapter 6 Support Squad

1. Brené Brown, *Daring Greatly: How the Courage to Be Vulnerable Transforms the Way We Live, Love, Parent, and Lead* (Gotham Books, 2012), 8.

2. *Our Epidemic of Loneliness and Isolation: The U.S. Surgeon General's Advisory on the Healing Effects of Social Connection and Community*, US Department of Health and Human Services, 2023, https://pubmed.ncbi.nlm.nih.gov/37792968/.

3. Machell Town et al., "Racial and Ethnic Differences in Social Determinants of Health and Health-Related Social Needs Among Adults—Behavioral Risk Factor Surveillance System, United States, 2022," *Morbidity and Mortality Weekly Report* 73, no. 9 (2024): 204–8.

4. "Risk Factors," *Centers for Disease Control and Prevention*, May 15, 2024, https://www.cdc.gov/social-connectedness/risk-factors/index.html.

5. April Simpkins and Cheslie Kryst, *By the Time You Read This* (Forefront Books, 2024).

6. Portia Jackson Preston et al., "'I Am Never Enough': Factors Contributing to Secondary Traumatic Stress and Burnout among Black Student Services Professionals in Higher Education," *Trauma Care* 3, no. 2 (2023): 93–107, https:// www.mdpi.com/2673-866X/3/2/10.

7. Oprah Winfrey, "When People Show You Who They Are, Believe Them," OWN Network, Oprah's Lifeclass, October 26, 2011, https://www.oprah.com /oprahs-lifeclass/when-people-show-you-who-they-are-believe-them-video.

8. Miguel R. Ramos et al., "Variety Is the Spice of Life: Diverse Social Networks Are Associated with Social Cohesion and Well-Being," *Psychological Science* 35, no. 6 (2024): 665–80.

## Chapter 7  Self-Preservation

1. Frank Pega et al., "Global, Regional, and National Burdens of Ischemic Heart Disease and Stroke Attributable to Exposure to Long Working Hours for 194 Countries, 2000–2016: A Systematic Analysis from the WHO/ILO Joint Estimates of the Work-Related Burden of Disease and Injury," *Environment International* 154 (2021), https://doi.org/10.1016/j.envint.2021.106595.

2. Christina Maslach and Michael P. Leiter, "Burnout," in *Stress: Concepts, Cognition, Emotion, and Behavior*, ed. George Fink (Elsevier Academic Press, 2016), 351–57.

3. Denise Albieri Jodas Salvagioni et al., "Physical, Psychological, and Occupational Consequences of Job Burnout: A Systematic Review of Prospective Studies," *PLOS ONE* 12, no. 10 (2017), https://doi.org/10.1371/journal.pone.0185781.

4. David S. Cross et al., "Understanding Pilots' Perceptions of Mental Health Issues: A Qualitative Phenomenological Investigation Among Airline Pilots in the United States," *Cureus* 16, no. 8 (August 2024), https://doi.org/10.7759/cureus.66277.

5. *2023 Work in America Survey*, American Psychological Association, https://www.apa.org/pubs/reports/work-in-america/2023-workplace-health-well-being.

6. *The U.S. Surgeon General's Framework for Workplace Mental Health & Well-Being*, US Department of Health and Human Services, 2022, https://www.hhs.gov/surgeongeneral/priorities/workplace-well-being/index.html.

## Chapter 8  Create Your Blueprint

1. Geoff Brumfiel, "Researchers Say Time Is an Illusion, So Why Are We All Obsessed with It?" *OPB*, December 28, 2022, https://www.opb.org/article/2022/12/28/researchers-say-time-is-an-illusion-so-why-are-we-all-obsessed-with-it.

2. Shailja Patel (@shailjapatelx), "'We all have the same 24 hours.' Use public transport? Your 24 hours are not the same as those of private jet owners. Do your own cooking, cleaning, child-raising? Your 24 hours are not the same as those of someone with a full-time domestic staff. Stop this nonsense," Twitter (now X), July 19, 2018, https://x.com/shailjapatel/status/1020158618350571520?lang=en.

3. Rose Horowitch, "The Elite College Students Who Can't Read Books," *The Atlantic*, October 1, 2024, https://www.theatlantic.com/magazine/archive/2024/11/the-elite-college-students-who-cant-read-books/679945/.

4. Portia Jackson Preston, "Break Free from the Shame Spiral," *Shame-Free Wellness*, February 10, 2025, https://portiajp.substack.com/p/break-free-from-the-shame-spiral.

## Chapter 9  Wellness Beyond Ourselves

1. Carl Honoré, *In Praise of Slowness: How a Worldwide Movement is Challenging the Cult of Speed* (HarperOne, 2004).

2. bell hooks, *Belonging: A Culture of Place* (Routledge, 2008) 223.

3. Desmond Tutu, interview with Tim Modise, Canonical Ltd., May 24, 2006, https://en.wikipedia.org/wiki/File:Experience_ubuntu.ogv.

4. Ben Sisario, "Jimmy Carter and Motown Founder Berry Gordy's Surprising Connection," *New York Times*, December 30, 2024, http://nytimes.com/2024/12/30/arts/music/jimmy-carter-berry-gordy.html.

5. Ryan Dunn, "Mr. Rogers' Words for Times of Tragedy," United Methodist Communications, August 7, 2019, https://www.umc.org/en/content/mr-rogers-words-for-times-of-tragedy.

**Portia Preston, DrPH**, is the founder and CEO of Empowered to Exhale, where she works with individuals and organizations to create a culture of sustainable wellness and performance. As an associate professor of public health at California State University, Fullerton, she focuses on inclusive approaches to wellness and creates innovative programming to support students, faculty, and staff. Portia holds a BA in cultural and social anthropology from Stanford University, a master of public health 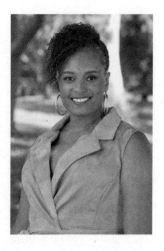 from the University of Michigan, and a doctorate of public health from UCLA. She lives in Long Beach, California.

## CONNECT WITH PORTIA

PortiaPreston.com

 DrPortiaPreston.Substack.com  @DrPortiaPreston

Dear Reader,

Thank you for selecting a Revell book! We're so happy to be part of your life through this work.

Revell's mission is to publish books that offer hope and help for meeting life's challenges, and that bring comfort and inspiration. We know that the right words at the right time can make all the difference; it is our goal with every title to provide just the words you need.

We believe in building lasting relationships with readers, and we'd love to get to know you better. If you have any feedback, questions, or just want to chat about your experience reading this book, please email us directly at publisher@revellbooks.com. Your insights are incredibly important to us, and it would be our pleasure to hear how we can better serve you.

We look forward to hearing from you and having the chance to enhance your experience with Revell Books.

The Publishing Team at Revell Books
A Division of Baker Publishing Group
publisher@revellbooks.com

Revell